CONCISE GUIDE TO

Women's Mental Health

American Psychiatric Press

CONCISE GUIDES

Robert E. Hales, M.D.
Series Editor

CONCISE GUIDE TO
Women's Mental Health

Vivien K. Burt, M.D., Ph.D.
Associate Professor of Clinical Psychiatry,
Department of Psychiatry and Biobehavioral Sciences
Director, Women's Life Center,
Neuropsychiatric Institute and Hospital
University of California at Los Angeles
Medical Director, Mental Health Clinic,
West Los Angeles Veterans Administration Medical Center
Los Angeles, California

Victoria C. Hendrick, M.D.
Assistant Clinical Professor of Psychiatry,
Department of Psychiatry and Biobehavioral Sciences,
University of California at Los Angeles
Edelman Westside Mental Health Center,
Los Angeles, California

American Psychiatric
Press, Inc.

Washington, DC
London, England

Copyright © 1997 American Psychiatric Press, Inc.
ALL RIGHTS RESERVED
Manufactured in the United States of America on acid-free paper
00 99 98 97   4 3 2 1

American Psychiatric Press, Inc.
1400 K Street, N.W., Washington, DC 20005

Library of Congress Cataloging-in-Publication Data

Burt, Vivien K., 1944-
    Concise guide to women's mental health / Vivien K. Burt and
Victoria C. Hendrick.
        p.   cm. — (Concise guides)
    Includes bibliographical references and index.
    ISBN 0-88048-343-1 (alk. paper)
    1. Gynecology—Psychological aspects.   2. Obstetrics—
Psychological aspects.   3. Women—Mental health.   I. Hendrick,
Victoria C., 1963-   .   II. Title.   III. Series: Concise guides
(American Psychiatric Press)
    [DNLM: 1. Mental Disorders. 2. Women—psychology. 3. Genital
Diseases, Female—psychology. 4. Women's Health. WA 309 B973c
1997]
RG103.5.B87 1997
616.89′0082—dc21
DNLM/DLC
for Library of Congress   96-45091
                                                                    CIP

British Library Cataloguing in Publication Data
A CIP record is available from the British Library.

To Josh, Kira, and Alex

CONTENTS

TABLES

FIGURES

INTRODUCTION

to the American Psychiatric Press Concise Guides

The American Psychiatric Press *Concise Guide* series provides practical information for psychiatrists, psychiatry residents, and medical students who work in a variety of treatment settings: inpatient psychiatry services, outpatient clinics, consultation-liaison services, and private practice. The *Concise Guides* are meant to complement the more detailed information to be found in lengthier psychiatry texts.

The *Concise Guides* address topics of special concern to psychiatrists in clinical practice. The books in this series contain a detailed table of contents, along with an index, tables, figures, and other charts for easy access. They are designed to fit into a lab coat pocket or jacket pocket, making them a convenient source of information. The number of references has been limited to those most relevant to the material presented.

Over the last several years, there has been increasing attention in psychiatric practice to the special needs of women. The authors of this *Concise Guide,* Drs. Vivien Burt and Victoria Hendrick, are experts in this burgeoning field. Both are on the faculty at the University of California at Los Angeles. Dr. Burt is the founder and director of the Women's Life Center at the UCLA Neuropsychiatric Institute and Hospital. A former physiology professor, Dr. Burt brings special expertise in molecular biology and physiology. Dr. Hendrick, one of her former residents and fellows, is now an attending in the Department of Psychiatry and Biobehavioral Sciences at the UCLA Neuropsychiatric Institute. Both authors have written extensively on many topics related to women's mental health and have extensive experience in the treatment of women patients at the Women's Life Center.

They begin their book by discussing important gender differences in the diagnosis of psychiatric disorders and in the psychopharmacological treatment of these conditions in women. In addition, they discuss important laboratory evaluation issues relevant to women and provide a concise outline of clinically significant considerations in the psychiatric assessment of women. The next nine chapters focus on important clinical conditions and psychiatric disorders found in women: premenstrual dysphoric disorder, hormonal contraception and effects on mood, psychiatric disorders in pregnancy, postpartum psychiatric disorders, elective abortion, infertility, perimenopause and menopause, gender issues in the treatment of major mental illness, and female-specific cancers.

The chapter on premenstrual dysphoric disorder focuses on the diagnosis and evaluation of this disorder in clinical practice. The authors also provide information on the differential diagnosis and the psychopharmacological and nonpsychopharmacological treatment of this condition. Their next chapter, on contraception, discusses risks and benefits of oral contraceptives and the relative contraindications to their use. In addition, the authors provide helpful information concerning the relative estrogenic, progestational, and androgenic activity of selected oral contraceptives.

In the chapter on pregnancy, the authors emphasize general principles that clinicians may consider in the management of pregnant patients with psychiatric disorders. The authors also provide helpful information on the U.S. Food and Drug Administration (FDA) pregnancy ratings for selected medications and summarize the in utero effects of common psychiatric medications. Also discussed are the relative risks and benefits of various treatments, including electroconvulsive therapy (ECT) in pregnant women, and the commonly reported teratogenic effects of abused drugs, including the fetal alcohol syndrome.

The chapter on postpartum psychiatric disorders begins by

providing epidemiological information concerning the incidence, time course, and clinical features of postpartum psychiatric disorders. The authors then discuss various treatment options for women with a postpartum psychiatric condition and provide useful information concerning the effects of selected psychotropic drugs in breast-feeding women.

The chapter on elective abortion contains practical clinical information about the psychological effects of abortion and about principles that practitioners may want to consider when counseling women who have undergone abortion. In their next chapter, on infertility, the authors provide an excellent overview for psychiatrists of current diagnostic studies used to evaluate infertility and discuss conventional infertility treatments, including relative success rates. Drs. Burt and Hendrick also provide helpful advice about the adverse effects of infertility and infertility procedures on women and their spouses and outline appropriate roles for psychiatrists in the collaborative management of patients undergoing infertility treatments.

The authors then turn their attention to the perimenopause and menopause. They discuss factors associated with the development of depression in the menopause transition and also the common doses and preparations of estrogen and progestin used to treat various physical symptoms that often occur in women during these periods. Their next chapter, on gender issues in the treatment of major mental illness, places special emphasis on schizophrenia, mood disorders, and substance abuse. They outline a number of important issues that should be considered by clinicians when treating these disorders in women.

The authors end their book by discussing breast cancer, gynecological cancer, and the role of psychiatric consultation to physicians treating women with these diseases.

Many excellent features make the book particularly outstanding for psychiatry residents, medical students, and psychiatric attendings who frequently treat women in their practices.

The authors have included more than 50 tables and figures, making the information readily available to clinicians, and there are a number of 1995–1997 references. Readers will find the clear, precise prose and clinically relevant information quite applicable to their practices. In this *Concise Guide,* the authors demonstrate both their remarkable ability to integrate complex material in a coherent and logical fashion and their significant clinical experience in treating women patients.

Drs. Burt and Hendrick have prepared an outstanding *Concise Guide to Women's Mental Health.* This wonderfully written pocket-sized book should be of great help to psychiatrists and other mental health professionals who treat women with psychiatric disorders.

Robert E. Hales, M.D.
Series Editor
American Psychiatric Press Concise Guide Series

PREFACE

This book is a practical guide to assessing and managing psychiatric conditions in women. It is derived from readings and seminars of the Women's Life Center at the UCLA Neuropsychiatric Institute and Hospital.

Increasingly, to ensure comprehensive psychiatric care for women patients, psychiatrists and other treating clinicians must maintain an ongoing knowledge of state-of-the-art advances in medicine, oncology, obstetrics, and gynecology. To support this effort, we review medical, obstetrical, and gynecological treatment modalities and their relevance to psychiatric illness in women. It is presumed that readers have a good understanding of the basic principles of psychiatric assessment, diagnosis, and treatment.

We also review the biological, psychological, and sociocultural factors influencing the mental health of women, with particular emphasis on reproductive points in the female life cycle. Finally, we review the ways in which these factors are relevant to differential diagnoses, case formulations, and treatment planning for women with psychiatric conditions. To crystallize the clinical information provided in the text, tables and figures are included. Many may be used for reference in practical clinical situations.

We would like to acknowledge the editorial comments of Ingrid Rodi, M.D., Josepha Seletz, M.D., and Carol Fred, M.S.W., and the technical assistance of Phyllis Davis. Additionally, we wish to thank Lori Altshuler, M.D., for her continued support in our endeavors. Finally, we thank the residents and fellows who have devoted themselves to the work of the Women's Life Center. It is through their energy, commitment, and determination that we were encouraged to write this guide to women's mental health.

Vivien K. Burt, M.D., Ph.D.
Victoria C. Hendrick, M.D.

INTRODUCTION

Women are the biggest consumers of health care in the United States. They make more visits than men to doctors' offices, fill more prescriptions, have more surgeries, occupy more than 60% of all hospital beds, and spend two out of every three health care dollars (1). During the 1980s and 1990s, the special health care needs of women have received increasing attention, leading to a better understanding of the psychiatric disorders to which they are vulnerable. This book is a guide to the assessment and management of psychiatric conditions specific to women.

■ GENDER DIFFERENCES IN PSYCHIATRIC DISORDERS

Gender differences in the prevalence of psychiatric disorders have long been recognized; prevalence rates in women exceed those of men for a number of disorders (2–4) (Table 1–1).

Gender-related differences exist not only in the lifetime prevalence of psychiatric disorders, but also in the expression, comorbidity, and course of many illnesses. For example, depression and dysthymia, both more common in women than in men, are more likely to be accompanied by anxiety disorders in women. Depressed women are more likely than are men to experience "atypical" symptoms, including hypersomnia and hyperphagia. Although bipolar disorder is about equally prevalent in both genders, women are more prone to rapid mood cycling. The course of schizophrenia is more favorable in women, who tend to have a later onset of the illness, fewer negative symptoms, and a better treatment response to the illness than do men.

Gender differences in psychiatric conditions may be due in part to psychosocial factors. Women's traditionally disadvantaged social status, lower wages, and increased vulnerability to sexual and domestic violence may contribute to their higher

TABLE 1–1. **Gender differences in lifetime prevalence of psychiatric disorders**

	Prevalence	
Disorder	Women	Men
Depression[a]	21.3	12.7
Dysthymia[a]	8.0	4.8
Bipolar disorder[b]		
Bipolar I	0.9	0.7
Bipolar II	0.5	0.4
Seasonal affective disorder[c]	6.3	1.0
Panic disorder[a]	5.0	2.0
Social phobia[a]	15.5	11.1
Generalized anxiety disorder[a]	6.6	3.6
Schizophrenia[b]	1.7	1.2
Alcohol dependence[a]	8.2	20.1
Alcohol abuse without dependence[a]	6.4	12.5
Drug dependence[b]	5.9	9.2
Drug abuse without dependence[b]	3.5	5.4
Anorexia nervosa[d,e]	0.5	0.05
Bulimia[f]	1.1	0.1
Antisocial personality[a]	1.2	5.8

Source. Data taken from following references:
[a]Kessler et al. 1994 (2).
[b]Weissman et al. 1991 (3).
[c]Rosenthal et al. 1984 (22).
[d]Walter and Kendler 1995 (20).
[e]Garfinkel 1995 (21).
[f]Garfinkel et al. 1995 (19).

rates of depressive and anxiety disorders. Biological gender differences may also explain some of the differences in psychiatric illnesses between men and women. Research is increasingly revealing that gender differences exist in brain anatomy and that male and female reproductive hormones have psychoactive effects (5,6). The psychoactive effects of estrogen and progesterone have received particular attention. Estrogen's antidopaminergic (7) and serotonin-enhancing (8) effects and modulation of γ-aminobutyric acid (GABA) receptors by metabolites of progesterone (9) may play a role in psychiatric disorders in women.

■ GENDER DIFFERENCES IN PSYCHOPHARMACOLOGY

Increasing data show that gender differences exist in the pharmacokinetics and pharmacodynamics of medications. Gender differences have been noted in rates of hepatic metabolism (10, 11), possibly due to estrogen's inhibitory effect on some hepatic microsomal enzymes (10, 12). Progesterone, by delaying gastric emptying time, may influence drug absorption. Estrogen and progesterone, both highly protein-bound, may compete with psychotropic medications for protein binding sites. Free, unbound levels of medications may thus vary with reproductive hormone levels. However, the net influence of physiological levels of reproductive hormones on drug metabolism is unclear. Because these hormones may induce some steps in hepatic metabolism while inhibiting others (13), the pharmacological effects of reproductive hormones are complex and poorly understood.

The effect of the menstrual cycle on psychotropic medication levels is unclear, although case reports suggest that levels may vary across the cycle (14–16). The use of exogenous hormones (e.g., oral contraceptives or hormone replacement therapy) may additionally influence levels of medications. Exogenous hormones inhibit oxidative hepatic metabolism, thus increasing blood levels of drugs that are oxidatively metabolized (e.g., many tricyclic antidepressants, diazepam, clonazepam, chlordiazepoxide). Oral contraceptives appear to induce hepatic conjugative enzymes, thus increasing clearance of drugs that are conjugated before elimination by the kidney (e.g., lorazepam, oxazepam, temazepam).

■ LABORATORY EVALUATION: SIGNIFICANT CONSIDERATIONS FOR WOMEN

Certain laboratory data are important parts of the workup of women patients. For example, since thyroid disorders are not uncommon in women, especially those older than 40, a full thyroid panel should be obtained in women reporting changes in energy level, weight, or temperature tolerance. For middle-aged women, follicle-stimulating hormone (FSH) and estradiol levels may be helpful in identifying perimenopausal and menopausal status. Pregnancy should be ruled out if psychotropic medications are to be initiated, particularly in women who have had unprotected intercourse or who have recently missed their menstrual period. A pregnancy test registers positive 10–14 days after conception. Commercially available pregnancy tests are simple to use and provide results within 5 minutes. They are 98% accurate, whereas blood tests for β-human chorionic gonadotropin (β-HCG) are 99%–100% accurate.

If a woman reports irregular or absent menses, a prolactin level and thyroid-stimulating hormone (TSH) level should be obtained, as both hyperprolactinemia and hypothyroidism may influence menstrual patterns. Hyperprolactinemia, a common side effect of neuroleptic medication, may require endocrinological consultation and brain imaging to rule out a prolactin-producing pituitary tumor. For women with a history of an eating disorder, albumin, total protein, and glucose levels can help assess nutritional status; amylase levels give an indication of the extent of self-induced vomiting; electrolytes, blood urea nitrogen, and creatinine levels are essential for assessing fluid and electrolyte abnormalities. A complete blood count can reveal anemia from nutritional deficiency and from internal bleeding—for example, from esophageal tears resulting from self-induced vomiting. An electrocardiogram should be obtained, because cardiac conduction abnormalities may occur as a result of electrolyte imbalance, malnutrition, and ipecac-induced cardiomyopathy.

■ THE PSYCHIATRIC ASSESSMENT OF WOMEN

Gender-specific aspects of the psychiatric assessment of women are summarized in Table 1–2. Clinicians should be alert to the elements of the history that are specifically relevant to women patients. For example, it is important to assess the relationship of the patient's symptoms to her menstrual cycle, to inquire about the possibility that she may be pregnant, and to ask about her use of contraception. The clinician should also ask about the patient's plans regarding pregnancy, because they may influence the choice of treatment (e.g., pharmacotherapy versus psychotherapy). In a middle-aged woman reporting sleep impairment, it is important to consider that perimenopausal night sweats may be disrupting her sleep. Seasonality of mood symptoms should be explored, because seasonal affective disorder predominates in women.

Because reproduction-related mood symptoms often run in families, a family history of premenstrual dysphoric disorder and depression should be obtained. Women with histories of sexually transmitted illnesses may be left with residual anger, guilt, or sadness because they are unable to conceive or retain a pregnancy. They may experience recurrent gynecological conditions (e.g., genital warts, genital herpes) that affect their sexual functioning. Breast surgery and hysterectomy may influ-

TABLE 1–2. **Psychiatric assessment of women: clinically significant considerations**

Component	Consideration
History of present illness and past psychiatric history	Characterize symptoms in relation to 1. A specific phase of the menstrual cycle 2. Use of hormonal contraception 3. Pregnancy 4. The postpartum period 5. Breast-feeding or weaning 6. Abortion 7. Infertility treatment 8. Hysterectomy 9. Perimenopause
Medications	Include exogenous hormones (oral or injectable contraceptives, postmenopausal hormone replacement, fertility medications) and all over-the-counter medications.
Dietary assessment	Rule out ritualistic or restrictive eating patterns, bingeing, self-induced vomiting, use of diet pills, laxatives, emetics, diuretics.
Alcohol and drugs	Rule out covert use, especially of prescription medications.
Family psychiatric history	Include history in female family members of premenstrual dysphoric disorder, postpartum mood disorders.
Medical history	Rule out autoimmune illnesses (e.g., lupus, thyroiditis, fibromyalgia) that may present with psychiatric symptoms. Rule out history of sexually transmitted disease that may affect current sexual functioning and childbearing capacity.
Menstrual history	Rule out pregnancy, menstruation-related symptoms (e.g., bloating, weight gain, cramping, breast tenderness). Rule out perimenopausal symptoms (e.g., irregular menstrual periods, hot flashes).

(continued)

TABLE 1–2. **Psychiatric assessment of women: clinically significant considerations** *(continued)*

Component	Consideration
Social and developmental history	Note sexual preference, relationship styles, level of satisfaction with current relationships. Document tendency to take on certain roles in relationships (e.g., as caregiver, nurturer, or as dependent or helpless).
	Note current or past sexual, physical, or emotional abuse.
Socioeconomic status	Note level of economic support and ability to meet ongoing financial needs. If patient is a single mother, inquire about child support.

ence a woman's sense of femininity and sexuality and may affect her relationship with her partner. Alcohol and drug abuse, although less prevalent in women than men, are a significant problem for some women (see Chapter 9). Women with a history of psychiatric symptoms occurring in relation to one reproductive life event (e.g., the use of oral contraceptives, premenstrually, postpartum, or perimenopausally) are at risk for the development of psychiatric symptoms at the time of subsequent reproductive life events (17).

Treating clinicians should also be aware of the social roles and pressures that may influence a woman's coping capacity and vulnerability to psychopathology. Economic conditions frequently dictate access to health care in general and to mental health care in particular. The greater number of female-headed households and the lower salaries for women than men continue to place increasing economic stress on women. Elderly women are particularly affected by economic difficulties. As they live longer, their increased risk of illness further stresses their financial resources (18). A woman may need encouragement to discuss strains in her life, such as family or marital conflict, domestic violence, or exhausting caretaking responsibilities, because she may feel guilty or disloyal about voicing her own needs when they conflict with those of family members.

■ REFERENCES

1. Collins JB: Women and the health care system, in Women's Health: A Primary Guide. Edited by Youngkin EQ, Davis MS. Norwalk, CT, Appleton & Lange, 1994, pp 5–6

2. Kessler RC, McGonagle KA, Zhao S, et al: Lifetime and 12-month prevalence of DSM-III-R psychiatric disorders in the United States: results from the National Comorbidity Survey. Arch Gen Psychiatry 51:8–19, 1994

3. Weissman MM, Livingston MB, Leaf PJ, et al: Affective disorders, in Psychiatric Disorders in America: The Epidemiologic Catchment Area Study. New York, Free Press, 1991, pp 53–80

4. Parry B: Reproductive factors affecting the course of affective illness in women, in Psychiatric Clinics of North America, Vol. 12. Edited by Parry B. Philadelphia, PA, WB Saunders, 1989, pp 221–230

5. McGlone J: Sex differences in human brain asymmetry: a critical survey. Behavioral and Brain Sciences 3:215–263, 1980

6. Vogel W, Klaiber EL, Broverman DM: The role of gonadal steroid hormones in psychiatric depression in men and women. Progress in Neuro-Psychopharmacology 2:487–503, 1978

7. Seeman MV, Lang M: The role of estrogens in schizophrenia gender differences. Schizophr Bull 16:185–194, 1990

8. Sherwin BB: Up-regulatory effect of estrogen on platelet 3H-imipramine binding sites in surgically menopausal women. Biol Psychiatry 28:339–348, 1990

9. Freeman W, Purdy RH, Coutifaris C, et al: Anxiolytic metabolites of progesterone: correlation with mood and performance measures following oral progesterone administration to healthy female volunteers. Clinical Neuroendocrinology 58:478–484, 1993

10. Hendrick V, Altshuler LL, Burt VK: Course of psychiatric disorders across the menstrual cycle. Harvard Review of Psychiatry 4:200–207, 1996

11. Greenblatt DJ, Allen MD, Harmatz JS, et al: Diazepam disposition determinants. Clin Pharmacol Ther 27:301–312, 1980

12. Fazio A: Oral contraceptive drug interactions: important considerations. South Med J 84:997–1002, 1991

13. Yonkers KA, Hamilton JA: Psychotropic medications, in Review of Psychiatry, Vol. 14. Edited by Oldham JM, Riba MB. Washington, DC, American Psychiatric Press, 1995, pp 307–332

14. Kimmel S, Gonsalves L, Youngs D, et al: Fluctuating levels of antidepressants. Journal of Psychosomatic Obstetrics and Gynecology 2:109–115, 1992

15. Conrad CD, Hamilton JA: Recurrent premenstrual decline in lithium concentration: clinical correlates and treatment implications. J Am Acad Child Adolesc Psychiatry 26:852–853, 1986

16. Kukopulos A, Minnai G, Muller-Oerlinghausen B: The influence of mania and depression on the pharmacokinetics of lithium. J Affect Disord 8:159–166, 1985

17. Stewart DE, Boydell KM: Psychologic distress during menopause: associations across the reproductive life cycle. Int J Psychiatry Med 23:157–162, 1993

18. Collins JB: Women and the health care system, in Women's Health: A Primary Guide. Edited by Youngkin EQ, Davis MS. Norwalk, CT, Appleton & Lange, 1994, p 30

■ FURTHER READINGS

Garfinkel PE: Eating disorders, in Comprehensive Textbook of Psychiatry, Sixth Edition. Edited by Kaplan HI, Sadock BJ. Baltimore, Williams & Wilkins, 1995, p 1364

Garfinkel PE, Lin E, Goering P, et al: Bulimia nervosa in a Canadian community sample: prevalence and comparison of subgroups. Am J Psychiatry 152:1052–1058, 1995

Rosenthal NE, Sack DA, Gillin JC, et al: Seasonal affective disorder: a description of the syndrome and preliminary findings with light therapy. Arch Gen Psychiatry 41:72–80, 1984

Walter EE, Kendler KS: Anorexia nervosa and anorexia-like syndromes in a population-based female twin sample. Am J Psychiatry 152:64–71, 1995

2

PREMENSTRUAL DYSPHORIC DISORDER

In DSM-IV (1), the diagnosis of premenstrual dysphoric disorder (PMDD) has been introduced under mood disorders not otherwise classified and replaces the previously named late luteal phase dysphoric disorder (LLPDD). It describes recurrent physical and emotional symptoms that occur in the last week of the menstrual cycle and remit within a day or two following onset of menstruation. Criteria for PMDD are listed in Table 2–1 (1). Notably, because of the poor reliability of retrospective reports, the diagnosis is made prospectively over at least two consecutive cycles. Nevertheless, in clinical practice, a provisional diagnosis is often made before confirmation through prospective ratings. Prospective ratings are made with a chart such as that shown in Figure 2–1. Although many women experience premenstrual somatic and psychological symptoms, only 5% have symptoms severe enough to meet criteria for PMDD.

■ ETIOLOGY

A number of etiologies have been suggested for PMDD. They include abnormal levels of estrogen, progesterone, follicle-stimulating hormone (FSH), luteinizing hormone (LH), cortisol, dihydrotestosterone, thyroid hormones, endogenous

TABLE 2–1. **DSM-IV criteria for premenstrual dysphoric disorder**

A. In most menstrual cycles during the past year, five (or more) of the following symptoms were present for most of the time during the last week of the luteal phase, began to remit within a few days after the onset of the follicular phase, and were absent in the week postmenses, with at least one of the symptoms being either (1), (2), (3), or (4):

   (1) markedly depressed mood, feelings of hopelessness, or self-deprecating thoughts
   (2) marked anxiety, tension, feelings of being "keyed up," or "on edge"
   (3) marked affective lability (e.g., feeling suddenly sad or tearful or increased sensitivity to rejection)
   (4) persistent and marked anger or irritability or increased interpersonal conflicts
   (5) decreased interest in usual activities (e.g., work, school, friends, hobbies)
   (6) subjective sense of difficulty in concentrating
   (7) lethargy, easy fatigability, or marked lack of energy
   (8) marked change in appetite, overeating, or specific food cravings
   (9) hypersomnia or insomnia
   (10) a subjective sense of being overwhelmed or out of control
   (11) other physical symptoms, such as breast tenderness or swelling, headaches, joint or muscle pain, a sensation of "bloating," weight gain

B. The disturbance markedly interferes with work or school or with usual social activities and relationships with others (e.g., avoidance of social activities, decreased productivity and efficiency at work or school).

C. The disturbance is not merely an exacerbation of the symptoms of another disorder, such as major depressive disorder, panic disorder, dysthymic disorder, or a personality disorder (although it may be superimposed on any of these disorders).

(continued)

TABLE 2–1.   **DSM-IV criteria for premenstrual dysphoric disorder**   *(continued)*

D. Criteria A, B, and C must be confirmed by prospective daily ratings during at least two consecutive symptomatic cycles. (The diagnosis may be made provisionally prior to this confirmation.)

Note: In menstruating females, the luteal phase corresponds to the period between ovulation and the onset of menses, and the follicular phase begins with menses. In nonmenstruating females (e.g., those who have had a hysterectomy), the timing of luteal and follicular phases may require measurement of circulating reproductive hormones.

Source.   Reprinted from American Psychiatric Association: *Diagnostic and Statistical Manual of Mental Disorders, 4th Edition.* Washington, DC, American Psychiatric Association, 1994, pp 717–718. Copyright 1994, American Psychiatric Association. Used with permission.

---

opioids, and serotonin (2). Despite extensive research, however, no consistent etiology has been identified. The biological changes of the menstrual cycle probably play a significant role, because symptoms do not occur in the absence of menstrual cycling—e.g., before puberty, during pregnancy, or following menopause.

■ RISK FACTORS

Women with a history of postpartum depression and mood changes induced by oral contraceptives appear to be at increased risk for PMDD. A history of non–reproductive-related clinical depression also appears to be a risk factor, as does a family history of PMDD (3).

■ EVALUATION

The components of the evaluation for PMDD are listed in Table 2–2. Frequently, women presenting for treatment of what

14

MONTH: _____

None 0   Mild 1   1. Circle days of period   2. Chart severity of symptoms as follows:
                    Moderate 2   Severe 3

SYMPTOMS	1	2	3	4	5	6	7	8	9	10	11	12	13	14	15

SYMPTOMS	16	17	18	19	20	21	22	23	24	25	26	27	28	29	30

FIGURE 2–1.   Prospective daily rating chart for premenstrual dysphoric disorder.

they believe to be PMDD have instead another psychiatric disorder—for example, depression, dysthymia, or an anxiety disorder, possibly with premenstrual exacerbation (6). To screen for other psychiatric disorders, a careful psychiatric history and prospective evaluation are important. A medical history and a physical examination, including a pelvic examination, are also necessary in order to rule out disorders that may present with premenstrual symptoms, such as migraine, endometriosis, epilepsy, systemic lupus erythematosus, fibromyalgia, thyroid disorders, fibrocystic breast disease, and irritable bowel syndrome (see Table 2–3).

Although no specific laboratory tests to screen for PMDD exist, laboratory measures can help to exclude other disorders. If a patient reports lethargy or fatigue, thyroid function tests and a complete blood count should be obtained to rule out hypothyroidism or anemia. Prolactin and thyroid studies should be assessed if a patient reports irregular menstrual bleeding or amenorrhea. In women older than 40 who report irregular menstrual bleeding or hot flashes, FSH and estradiol levels should be measured.

Because diets high in caffeine, salt, and alcohol may worsen PMDD, a nutritional assessment can be useful. The patient should also be asked about her use of hormonal contraception, as both oral and injectable forms of contraception may induce mood changes.

■ TREATMENT STRATEGIES

Nonpharmacological Treatments

Reassurance and support should be offered to all women with PMDD. Educating the patient and her family about her premenstrual symptoms can help reduce feelings of shame, guilt, and helplessness. The daily routine of prospective ratings may give a woman a greater sense of predictability and control of

TABLE 2–2. **Evaluation of premenstrual dysphoric disorder**

Type of evaluation	Components
Psychiatric evaluation	History of symptoms, including duration, course, precipitating factors, and previous treatments and response
	Past psychiatric history, particularly of mood disorders
	History of alcohol and substance abuse
Medical evaluation	Medical history, including assessment of endocrine and gynecological disorders (e.g., thyroid abnormalities, endometriosis, fibrocystic breast disease)
Laboratory tests	Complete blood count and chemistry panel, including glucose, calcium, and magnesium; thyroid function tests
Family history	History of premenstrual symptoms, treatment strategies, and outcome in female relatives
Medication use	Assessment of medications that may produce psychiatric side effects (e.g., antihypertensive medications, bronchodilators, antiulcer agents, corticosteroids, analgesics, sedatives, decongestants)
Nutritional assessment	Assessment of use of caffeine, salt, alcohol; rule out potential nutritional deficiencies (e.g., vitamin B_6, calcium, magnesium)

her symptoms and may encourage her to rearrange her schedule to minimize stress during the premenstrual week. For women with mild premenstrual symptoms, nonpharmacological interventions may suffice and should be tried before beginning a medication trial (Table 2–4). The patient should be encouraged, for example, to get adequate sleep during her premenstrual week and to minimize her use of caffeine, salt, alcohol, and nicotine. Exercise, relaxation therapy, and cognitive-behavior therapy may also reduce symptoms (3). These nonpharmacological interventions may also be useful in ameliorating premenstrual symptoms while the patient's diagnosis is established through two monthly prospective ratings. If the patient's premenstrual symptoms developed or worsened following initiation of an oral contraceptive, a switch to another preparation or an alternative form of birth control may be helpful.

TABLE 2–3. **Medical differential diagnosis of premenstrual dysphoric disorder**

Endometriosis
Chronic fatigue syndrome
Migraine
Systemic lupus erythematosus
Irritable bowel syndrome
Epilepsy
Thyroid disorders
Fibrocystic breast disease

TABLE 2–4. **Nonpharmacological treatment strategies for premenstrual dysphoric disorder**

Education, support
Family intervention
Stress reduction
Dietary changes: reduce salt, alcohol, caffeine
Reduce or discontinue nicotine
Cognitive-behavioral approaches
Exercise
Relaxation techniques

Pharmacological Treatments

A wide variety of pharmacological treatments have been reported to reduce symptoms of PMDD (Table 2–5). Treatments generally use one of three strategies: symptom relief, modification of a possible biochemical imbalance, and suppression of ovulation.

Psychotropic treatments. Several controlled studies show that fluoxetine at 20 mg/day is effective for premenstrual dysphoria, irritability, and tension (3, 4). Other serotonergic medications, including paroxetine, sertraline, and clomipramine, also appear to treat premenstrual depression and anxiety successfully. To be effective, the antidepressants should be given throughout the menstrual cycle, although some success has been reported when fluoxetine is taken only during the 12–14 premenstrual days.

Nortriptyline and nefazodone at standard doses also appear to be helpful. For women with premenstrual anxiety and irritability, alprazolam and buspirone are reasonable choices. Alprazolam should be reserved only for patients without histories of substance abuse and should be tapered after the onset of menses. Dextroamphetamine has been reported to improve premenstrual lethargy, poor concentration, and hyperphagia when used during symptomatic days.

Hormonal strategies. Hormonal therapies are based on the premise that premenstrual symptoms result from the endocrine changes of the menstrual cycle. The drop in progesterone during the luteal phase (second half) of the menstrual cycle has been implicated as etiological in PMDD (Figure 2–2). Progesterone supplementation has been reported to reduce premenstrual symptoms and is currently the most widely used hormonal treatment. However, double-blind studies have failed to show the efficacy of either natural or synthetic progesterone

TABLE 2–5. **Pharmacological treatments for premenstrual dysphoric disorder**

Medication	Dosage	When administered
Psychotropic		
fluoxetine	20 mg qd	Throughout cycle
sertraline	50–100 mg qd	Throughout cycle
paroxetine	10–30 mg qd	Throughout cycle
clomipramine	25–75 mg qd	Throughout cycle
nortriptyline	50–100 mg qd	Throughout cycle
nefazodone	100–600 mg qd	Throughout cycle
dextroamphetamine	10–20 mg qd	During symptomatic days
alprazolam	0.25–5 mg qd	During symptomatic days
buspirone	15–60 mg qd	Throughout cycle or during symptomatic days
Nonpsychotropic		
estradiol		
Implants	50–100 mg subcutaneously	Every 4–7 months
Patches	2 patches at 100 µg	Every 3 days throughout cycle
gonadotropin-releasing hormone (GnRH) agonist		
leuprolide	3.75 mg intramuscularly	Every 4 weeks
danazol	200–400 mg	Daily from onset of symptoms to first day of menses
Diuretics		
spironolactone	25 mg qd–qid	During symptomatic days
hydrochlorothiazide	25–50 mg qd	During symptomatic days
Dyazide	1 capsule	During symptomatic days
Prostaglandin inhibitors		
ibuprofen	600 mg bid–tid	During symptomatic days
mefenamic acid	250–500 mg tid	During symptomatic days
naproxen sodium	500 mg qd–bid	During symptomatic days

(continued)

TABLE 2–5. **Pharmacological treatments for premenstrual dysphoric disorder** *(continued)*

Medication	Dosage	When administered
Vitamins/minerals		
Vitamin E	400 IU qd	Throughout cycle
pyridoxine	50–100 mg	Throughout cycle
calcium	500 mg bid	Throughout cycle
magnesium	360 mg qd–tid	Midcycle to onset of menses
bromocriptine	2.5 mg bid–tid	Day 10 to onset of menses
Evening primrose oil	1–4 gm	Throughout cycle or from midcycle to onset of menses
Antihypertensives		
clonidine	17 mcg/kg qd	Throughout cycle
atenolol	50 mg qd	Throughout cycle
naltrexone	25 mg bid	Days 9–18 of cycle

(3). Estrogen, prescribed either subcutaneously or transdermally, has been reported to treat premenstrual psychological and physical symptoms effectively (3). Side effects include nausea, breast tenderness, and weight gain. For reasons that are unclear, orally administered estrogen does not appear effective.

Danazol, a synthetic androgen, suppresses the hypothalamic-pituitary-ovarian axis, thus producing an anovulatory state. It has been reported to reduce premenstrual depression, irritability, edema, anxiety, and breast tenderness. Side effects, which are significant, include acne, weight gain, and hirsutism.

Similar symptomatic relief has been reported with gonadotropin-releasing hormone (GnRH) agonists such as leuprolide. Like danazol, GnRH agonists produce anovulation; both danazol and GnRH agonists cause estrogen to fall to menopausal levels, with the accompanying risks of osteoporosis, heart disease, hot flashes, and other symptoms of hypoestrogenemia. Until more data exist on the safety of these medications in

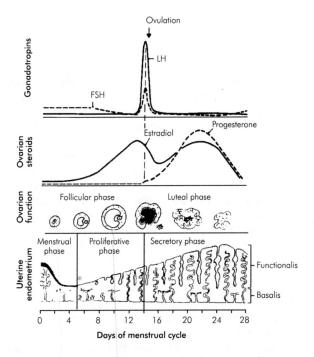

FIGURE 2–2. **Hormonal fluctuations across the menstrual cycle.** *Source.* Reprinted from Toot PJ, Surrey ES, Lu JKH: *Essentials of Obstetrics and Gynecology,* 2nd Edition. Edited by Hacker NF, Moore JG. Philadelphia, PA, W. B. Saunders, 1992, p. 39. Used with permission.

long-term use, they should not be considered a first-line treatment for the symptoms of PMDD.

Vitamins and minerals. Pyridoxine (vitamin B_6), a cofactor in the synthesis of dopamine and serotonin, appears to reduce depression, irritability, fatigue, edema, and headache at a dose of 50 mg/day. Patients should be warned not to use pyridoxine excessively, because doses above 100 mg/day have been associated with peripheral neuropathy.

Calcium, magnesium, and vitamin E have been tried for premenstrual depression, pain, and fatigue. Although data on their efficacy are mixed, these interventions are worth trying, as they are safe and generally well tolerated.

Diuretics.   For women with premenstrual fluid retention, diuretics may be of benefit. Spironolactone and Dyazide, a combination of hydrochlorothiazide and triamterene, help reduce not only premenstrual edema but also premenstrual dysphoria in women who experience diuresis. Hypokalemia, dizziness, and orthostasis are potential side effects. Women who do not experience premenstrual edema do not appear to benefit from diuretics.

Prostaglandin inhibitors.   Because prostaglandins modulate inflammatory responses and increase pain sensitivity, prostaglandin inhibitors can help reduce pain and swelling. In particular, mefenamic acid (Ponstel) and naproxen sodium (Anaprox, Naprosyn) are effective for premenstrual pelvic pain, cramping, and headache. For maximal efficacy, they should be started before the onset of symptoms—7–10 days prior to menstruation. The prostaglandin inhibitors do not appear effective, however, for premenstrual mood symptoms.

Other agents.   A variety of miscellaneous medications have been reported to reduce premenstrual symptoms. The β-blocker atenolol may improve premenstrual irritability, and the antihypertensive agent clonidine has been reported to relieve premenstrual anxiety, depression, hostility, and irritability. The opiate antagonist naltrexone may reduce general premenstrual symptoms, including irritability, anxiety, depression, lethargy, bloating, and headaches. For premenstrual mastalgia, the dopamine agonist bromocriptine is helpful and may also reduce premenstrual irritability, depression, and anxiety. Women should be advised to take bromocriptine with food, because it may cause nausea. Evening primrose oil, obtained over the counter in health food stores, has been noted to alleviate premenstrual mood symptoms.

■ APPROACH TO TREATMENT

Before treatment is begun, prospective daily symptom ratings should be obtained to confirm the diagnosis. Psychiatric and medical evaluations should exclude other disorders. Once the diagnosis has been made, simple interventions—for example, exercise, dietary modification, education, and stress reduction—should be encouraged for all patients, even when the decision has been made to initiate pharmacotherapy. In choosing among the various medications, important considerations include the patient's symptom profile and severity, her preference regarding treatment schedule (continuous or during symptomatic periods only), and the medication's side effects and addictive potential.

For patients with mild premenstrual depressive symptoms, vitamins, minerals, evening primrose oil, or a diuretic may be tried. They have the advantage of being well tolerated and need to be taken for only part of the cycle.

For patients with more severe premenstrual depression, a psychotropic drug or hormonal agent should be considered. The anxiolytics alprazolam and buspirone are helpful for premenstrual anxiety. A medication trial should extend for a minimum of two or three menstrual cycles to assess for efficacy.

Medications that suppress ovulation should not be used as first-line options, because little is known about their safety in prolonged use. Because they induce a hypoestrogenic state, they may increase the risk of osteoporosis and cardiovascular disease. Some researchers have suggested that long-term use of GnRH agonists may be safe if supplemented with estrogen and a progestin (3).

For patients with premenstrual symptoms that are refractory to the current treatment strategies, a lasting response has been reported with ovariectomy (5). Because this approach produces surgical menopause, estrogen supplementation is necessary. Clearly, this approach is drastic and should not be considered until other treatment strategies have been systematically and exhaustively explored.

Continuation of daily symptom ratings during treatment will allow assessment of symptomatic improvement and may help the patient gain a sense of control over her symptoms by visualizing their timing and predictability.

■ REFERENCES

1. American Psychiatric Association: Diagnostic and Statistical Manual of Mental Disorders, 4th Edition. Washington, DC, American Psychiatric Association, 1995, pp 717–718
2. Rubinow DR, Hoban MC, Grover GN, et al: Changes in plasma hormones across the menstrual cycle in patients with menstrually related mood disorder and control subjects. Am J Obstet Gynecol 158:5–11, 1988
3. Altshuler LL, Hendrick V, Parry B: Pharmacologic management of premenstrual disorder. Harvard Review of Psychiatry 2:223–245, 1995
4. Steiner M, Steinberg S, Stewart D, et al: Fluoxetine in the treatment of premenstrual dysphoria. N Engl J Med 332:1529–1534, 1995
5. Casson P, Hahn M, Van Vugt DA, et al: Lasting response to ovariectomy in severe intractable premenstrual syndrome. Am J Obstet Gynecol 162:99–105, 1990
6. Hendrick V, Altshuler LL, Burt VK: Course of psychiatric disorders across the menstrual cycle. Harvard Review of Psychiatry 4:200–207, 1996

HORMONAL CONTRACEPTION AND EFFECTS ON MOOD 3

■ HORMONAL CONTRACEPTION

The birth control pill is a popular form of contraception for women in their reproductive years. It is easy to use, and, when taken as prescribed, its efficacy rate (> 99%) is superior to alternative forms of contraception (Table 3–1).

Other advantages of oral contraceptives include regular menses and reduction of the risks of endometrial and ovarian cancer, ovarian cysts, ectopic pregnancy, and iron deficiency anemia (Table 3–2). Because of rare risks associated with their use (e.g., thrombovascular disease, hepatic tumors), oral contraceptives are contraindicated in women with certain conditions (Table 3–3). A large variety of formulations are currently on the market, falling into two main categories: combination pills (combining an estrogen and progestin) and progestin only. Combination pills are further categorized as monophasic (containing fixed doses of estrogen and progestin throughout the cycle) and as biphasic or triphasic (containing varying doses of hormone at different times of the cycle) (Table 3–4).

Brands of combination pills vary in their estrogenic, progestational, and androgenic activity (Table 3–5). In general, estrogenic side effects include nausea, breast tenderness, cystic breast changes, headaches, elevated blood pressure, and in-

TABLE 3–1.   Failure rates of various forms of contraception

Form of contraception	Failure rate	
	Typical use (%)	Perfect use (%)
No method	85	NA
Spermicide alone	21	6
Cervical cap with spermicide	18	11.5
Diaphragm with spermicide	18	6
Condom (male)	12	3
Condom (female)	21	5
Oral contraceptives		
Combined	3	0.1
Progestin only	no data	0.5
Medroxyprogesterone acetate		
(Provera)	0.3	0.3
Levonorgestrel implants		
(Norplant)	0.09	0.09
Intrauterine device		
Progesterone T	2	1.5
Copper T 380A	0.8	0.6

Source. Adapted from "Choice of Contraceptives" 1995 (10).

TABLE 3–2.   Risks and benefits of oral contraceptives

Increased risk	Decreased risk
Thromboembolism[a]	Endometrial cancer
Cerebrovascular accidents[a]	Ovarian cancer
Hypertension[a]	Pelvic inflammatory disease
Gallstones	Fibrocystic breast disease
Benign hepatic tumors	Iron deficiency anemia
Postpill amenorrhea	

[a]Primarily in smokers over age 35.

crease in the size of fibroid tissue. Progestin side effects include weight gain, fatigue, decreased libido, and headaches. Androgenic effects include hirsutism, acne, and weight gain.

Compared with combination pills, progestin-only pills are less

TABLE 3–3. **Absolute contraindications to use of oral contraceptives**

History of thrombophlebitis or thromboembolic disorder

History of coronary artery disease or myocardial infarction

Known or suspected carcinoma of the breast

Known or suspected estrogen-dependent neoplasia, especially carcinoma of the endometrium

Undiagnosed genital bleeding

Markedly impaired liver function

Smoking, age greater than 35, and obesity

Known or suspected pregnancy

Congenital hyperlipidemia (estrogen increases risk of cardiovascular death in these patients)

Obstructive jaundice in pregnancy

Source. Adapted from Speroff et al. 1983 (11).

TABLE 3–4. **Hormonal forms of contraception**

Oral contraceptives

    Combination (i.e., with both an estrogen and a progestin component)

        Monophasic (hormone levels remain steady throughout the pill cycle); examples include Brevicon, Loestrin, Demulen

        Triphasic (hormone levels vary across the pill cycle, to simulate a normal menstrual cycle); examples include Ortho-Novum 7/7/7, Tri-Norinyl, Tri-Levlen

    Progestin only; examples include Ovrette, Nor-Q.D., Micronor

Depo-Provera (150-mg medroxyprogesterone acetate injection every 3 months)

Norplant (5-year levonorgestrel subdermal implant)

effective and may cause irregular bleeding. However, they are indicated for women who are breast-feeding or who have contraindications to estrogens (e.g., hypertension, breast cancer).

TABLE 3–5. Relative estrogenic, progestational, and androgenic activity of some oral contraceptives

Contraceptive	Activity		
	Estrogenic	Progestational	Androgenic
Brevicon	++	+	+
Demulen	+	++	+
Desogen	+	−	+/−
Jenest-28	++	+	+/−
Lo-Ovral	+	+	+/−
Loestrin 1.5/30	+	+++	+++
Loestrin 1/20	+	++	++
Ortho-Novum 7/7/7	++	+	+/−
Orthocept	+	+	+/−
Ovcon-35	++	+	+
Tri-Levlen	++	+	+/−
Triphasil	++	+	+/−

+++ = highest. ++ = high. + = medium.
+/− = low. − = no activity.

Two long-acting hormonal forms of contraception, levonorgestrel implants (Norplant) and medroxyprogesterone acetate injections (Depo-Provera), have increased in popularity in recent years because of ease of use and reversibility. Norplant is a subdermal implant that provides up to 5 years of contraception, and Depo-Provera is an injectable progestogenic agent administered every 3 months. Side effects of Norplant and Depo-Provera include menstrual irregularities, acne, and weight gain.

■ EFFECTS OF HORMONAL CONTRACEPTION ON MOOD

A number of studies have reported an association between oral contraceptive use and clinical depression. However, the majority of these studies involved high-dose oral contraceptives no longer in use. Controlled studies with the newer, low-dose birth control pills do not suggest an association with new-onset clinical depression and oral contraceptive use. There are reports, however, of recurrence of depression in women with a history of depression or of premenstrual mood changes (1, 2).

Whether less severe (subclinical) depressive symptomatology is associated with oral contraceptives is unclear (1–3). Some data suggest that the triphasic preparations may be particularly likely to induce mood changes (4), particularly in women with a history of premenstrual depression (5). For women who do experience mood changes with the birth control pill, supplementation with vitamin B_6 (25–50 mg) (6) may help, because oral contraceptives may produce a functional vitamin B_6 deficiency (6). Independent of adverse effects on mood, oral contraceptives may also reduce sexual interest (7). Contraceptives with high progestational activity (e.g., 1.5 mg norethindrone acetate) may cause fatigue and lethargy.

Alternatively, some women experience mood enhancement with oral contraceptives. Oral contraceptives have been anecdotally reported to reduce symptoms of premenstrual syndrome (PMS), but prospective data have failed to show consistently positive results regarding relief of premenstrual mood symptoms; however, premenstrual bloating and breast pain are ameliorated (7).

Depot medroxyprogesterone acetate (Depo-Provera) has been reported anecdotally to cause negative mood symptoms, but the single study assessing its effect on mood found little evidence that it caused depression (8). Norplant has been associated with new-onset depression and panic attacks that resolved 1 month after its removal (9).

In conclusion, women with new onset mood changes should be assessed for recent initiation of hormonal contraception. Particularly for women with a history of premenstrual changes or depression, precipitation of dysphoria by the contraceptive should be considered. Switching to another hormonal contraceptive or to an alternative method of birth control may lead to resolution of the affective symptoms.

■ REFERENCES

1. Kendler KS, Martin NS, Heath AC, et al: A twin study of the psychiatric side effects of oral contraceptives. J Nerv Ment Dis 176:153–160, 1988

2. Bancroft J, Sartorius N: The effects of oral contraceptives on well-being and sexuality. Oxford Review of Reproductive Biology 12:57–92, 1990

3. Parry BL, Rush AJ: Oral contraceptives and depressive symptomatology: biologic mechanisms. Compr Psychiatry 20:347–358, 1979

4. Bancroft J, Rennie D: The impact of oral contraceptives on the experience of perimenstrual mood, clumsiness, food craving and other symptoms. J Psychosom Res 37:195–202, 1993

5. Bancroft J, Sanders D, Warner P, et al: The effects of oral contraceptives on mood and sexuality: a comparison of triphasic and combined preparations. Journal of Psychosomatic Obstetrics and Gynecology 7:1–8, 1987

6. Winston F: Oral contraceptives, pyridoxine, and depression. Am J Psychiatry 130:1217–1221, 1973

7. Graham CA, Sherwin BB: A prospective treatment study of premenstrual symptoms using a triphasic oral contraceptive. J Psychosom Res 36:257–266, 1992

8. Westhoff C, Wieland D, Tiezzi L: Depression in users of depo-medroxyprogesterone acetate. Contraception 51:351–354, 1995

9. Wagner KD, Berenson AB: Norplant-associated major depression and panic disorder. J Clin Psychiatry 55:478–480, 1994

10. Choice of contraceptives. The Medical Letter 37:9–10, 1995

11. Speroff L, Glass RH, Kase NG: Clinical Gynecologic Endocrinology and Infertility. Baltimore, MD, Williams & Wilkins, 1983, pp 433–442

PSYCHIATRIC DISORDERS IN PREGNANCY

Psychiatric disorders in women occur most frequently during the age range of 18–45 years. Because these are the childbearing years, many women may experience the onset of a psychiatric illness during pregnancy. For women with preexisting psychiatric illness, little is known about the influence of pregnancy on the course of psychiatric disorders. Available data suggest, however, that pregnancy is not a time of emotional stability, as has been traditionally thought. Frequently, women with psychiatric histories or those who are currently experiencing psychiatric symptoms request consultation regarding pharmacological management during a future or current pregnancy (Table 4–1).

■ GENERAL PRINCIPLES

Patients with active psychiatric disorders during pregnancy require careful assessment and management. The goal of treatment is to maintain psychiatric stability while minimizing risks to the developing fetus (Table 4–2).

■ NONPHARMACOLOGICAL INTERVENTIONS

Women should be advised to discontinue caffeine, nicotine, and alcohol during pregnancy. Although sleep disturbance is common during a normal pregnancy, sleep deprivation exacerbates psychiatric symptoms; therefore, an attempt should be made to maximize the opportunity for adequate rest. Relaxation techniques, cognitive-behavior therapy, and psychotherapy can be very helpful for anxiety, and environmental interventions may help reduce psychosocial stressors. Whenever possible, the patient's partner should be included in the treatment planning and decision making. If the relationship between the expectant parents is conflictual, conjoint therapy should be strongly encouraged before the delivery. Peer groups for pregnant women, which are becoming increasingly avail-

---

TABLE 4–1. **Patients requiring perinatal consultation**

Patient who is psychiatrically ill during pregnancy

Patient taking psychotropic medication who discovers she is pregnant

Patient with a history of psychiatric illness who is planning to become pregnant

Patient with a history of psychiatric illness who is pregnant

---

TABLE 4–2. **Management of psychiatric disorders during pregnancy: general principles**

Planned pregnancy allows time to discuss treatment options and to switch, if necessary, to a medication that appears safer in pregnancy.

Goal of pharmacotherapy is not maximum control of symptoms, but rather reduction of symptoms that jeopardize the mother or the pregnancy.

Whenever possible, psychotherapy and psychosocial measures should take precedence over pharmacotherapy or electroconvulsive therapy (ECT).

All treatment recommendations should be discussed with patient, partner, and obstetrician. All discussions before and during pregnancy should be documented.

---

able, may provide the patient with emotional and practical support (Table 4–3).

■ PHARMACOLOGICAL INTERVENTIONS

Although, for some women, therapy and supportive psychosocial measures may suffice, more severely ill patients may require psychopharmacological intervention or electroconvulsive therapy (ECT). The decision to use a psychotropic agent in pregnancy always requires a careful weighing of risks and benefits. Whenever a treatment plan is made, the risk to the mother and to the fetus from both the psychiatric disorder and the treatment regimen must be considered. Discontinuation of medication may result in relapse, putting a psychiatrically ill woman at increased risk for poor nutrition, inadequate prenatal care, and substance abuse. When possible, an attempt should be made to avoid psychopharmacology during the first 12 weeks of gestation, because this is the time of most active organ development (Figure 4–1). When possible, medications should be tapered or discontinued for patients who discover they are pregnant while taking a psychotropic agent. When

---

TABLE 4–3. **Nonpharmacological treatment interventions for psychiatric disorders during pregnancy**

Elimination of caffeine, nicotine, and alcohol

Adequate sleep

Relaxation techniques

Cognitive-behavior therapy

Support groups

Education

Marital therapy when necessary

Reduction of psychosocial stressors

Close communication with obstetrical service

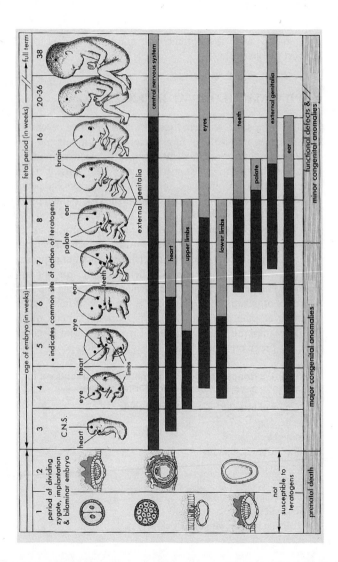

FIGURE 4-1. **Schematic illustration of the critical periods in human development.** During the first 2 weeks of life, the embryo is usually not susceptible to teratogens. During these preembryonic stages, a teratogen damages either all or most of the cells, resulting in death, or damages only a few cells, allowing the conceptus to recover and the embryo to develop without birth defects.
Bar graphs in figure: *Black,* highly sensitive periods of development when major defects may be produced (e.g., absence of limbs). *Gray,* stages that are less sensitive to teratogens, when minor defects may be induced (e.g., hypoplastic thumbs).
Source.   Reprinted from Moore KL, Persaud TVN: *The Developing Human: Clinically Oriented Embryology.* Philadelphia, PA, W. B. Saunders, 1993, p. 156. Used with permission.

medications are used during the first 2 gestational weeks (i.e., the period between conception and the first missed period), it is unlikely that the developing embryo will be exposed to them, because the uteroplacental circulation has not yet formed.

When a medication is used during pregnancy, the dosage should be maintained at the minimum necessary for control of symptoms. The aim is not so much to eliminate symptoms as to reduce them so that the patient is able to gain adequate weight and obtain appropriate prenatal care.

Before administering a psychotropic medication, the clinician should review with the patient, her obstetrician, and, when possible, her partner, all available data on the use of the medication during pregnancy. This review should include U.S. Food and Drug Administration (FDA) labeling for the medication (Table 4–4) (1). It is important to emphasize the limitations of current data, including limited sample sizes and confounding factors such as alcohol and substance abuse, maternal age, and diagnosis. Moreover, few studies have assessed potential neurobehavioral sequelae of prenatal medication exposure, a more subtle form of teratogenesis. Toward the end of pregnancy the pediatrician should be provided with information about potential neonatal sequelae of the medications used during pregnancy. All discussions should be carefully documented and should indicate the patient's capacity to consent to the treatment plan.

■ USE OF PSYCHOTROPIC MEDICATIONS DURING PREGNANCY

Table 4–5 summarizes the effects of in utero exposure to these types of medications.

Antidepressants

A relatively large literature on tricyclic antidepressants (TCAs) in pregnancy shows that they do not appear to increase the risk for congenital anomalies, even when used during the first trimester (2). They may, however, produce transient perinatal toxicity or withdrawal symptoms when used near delivery. Symptoms include jitteriness, irritability, lethargy, hypotonia, and anticholinergic effects such as constipation, tachycardia, and urinary retention (2).

Data on the use of selective serotonin reuptake inhibitors (SSRIs) during pregnancy are limited. The results of a small prospective study suggested that fluoxetine was not associated with a higher risk for congenital malformations when used in the first trimester (3). Although a single case report described

---

TABLE 4–4. U.S. Food and Drug Administration (FDA) use-in-pregnancy ratings

Rating	Interpretation
A	Controlled studies show no risk—adequate, well-controlled studies in pregnant women have failed to demonstrate risk to the fetus.
B	No evidence of risk in humans—either animal findings show risk, but human findings do not; or, if no adequate human studies have been done, animal findings are negative.
C	Risk cannot be ruled out—human studies are lacking, and animal studies are either positive for fetal risk or lacking as well; however, potential benefits may justify potential risk.
D	Positive evidence of risk—investigational or post-marketing data show risk to the fetus. Nevertheless, potential benefits may outweigh the potential risk.
X	Contraindicated in pregnancy—studies in animals or humans, or investigational or postmarketing reports, have shown fetal risks that clearly outweigh any possible benefit to the patient.

Source. Reprinted from *Physicians' Desk Reference* 1996 (1).

TABLE 4–5. Summary of in utero exposure to common psychotropic medications

Medication	Teratogenicity	Perinatal effects
Antidepressants		
Tricyclic and heterocyclic	Appear to be safe; nortriptyline and desipramine preferred	Toxicity and withdrawal symptoms include lethargy, hypotonia, jitteriness, irritability, anticholinergic effects (e.g., constipation, tachycardia, urinary retention)
SSRIs		
fluoxetine	No adverse effects (1 small study), probably safe	No clear data
sertraline	No clear data	No clear data
paroxetine	No clear data	No clear data
MAOIs	Contraindicated: increased rate of congenital anomalies in animal studies	Contraindicated: potential hypertensive crisis if tocolytic medications are needed
Other: bupropion, trazodone, venlafaxine, nefazodone	No clear data yet	No clear data yet

Mood stabilizers		
lithium	First-trimester exposure: approximately 0.01% risk of Ebstein's anomaly	Possible perinatal syndrome of hypotonia, poor suck reflex, hypoglycemia, cyanosis; reports of hypothyroidism, neonatal goiter, diabetes insipidus
carbamazepine	First-trimester exposure: 0.5%–1.0% risk of spina bifida; also developmental delay, craniofacial defects, fingernail hypoplasia	No clear data
valproic acid	First-trimester exposure: 1%–5% risk of spina bifida; also developmental delay, craniofacial defects, fingernail hypoplasia	No clear data
Antipsychotic agents	No general data; see specific categories below for data	Standard antipsychotic agents are associated with transient perinatal syndrome: restlessness, tremor, hypotonia, hyperreflexia, irritability, poor feeding
Low-potency	phenothiazines: small increase in non-specific congenital malformations	phenothiazines: reports of neonatal jaundice; cases of neonatal anticholinergic side effects noted

(continued)

TABLE 4–5. Summary of in utero exposure to common psychotropic medications (*continued*)

Medication	Teratogenicity	Perinatal effects
Antipsychotic agents (*continued*)		
High-potency	Appear safe	No clear data
clozapine	Single case: no adverse effects; more data needed	No data
risperidone	No data	No data
Benzodiazepines	Data mixed; some show increased risk of oral clefts (especially with diazepam, alprazolam); data on other teratogenic effects (e.g., growth retardation) controversial	With regular use in late pregnancy: transient perinatal toxicity syndrome (lethargy, hypothermia, hypotonia), withdrawal syndrome
Agents to treat antipsychotic side effects		
trihexyphenidyl	Minor congenital anomalies	Anticholinergic side effects
benztropine	Minor congenital anomalies	Anticholinergic side effects

diphenhydramine	Most studies suggest no increased risk of organ malformation	Neonatal withdrawal syndrome
amantadine	Cardiovascular malformations	No clear data

Note. MAOI = monoamine oxidase inhibitor. SSRI = selective serotonin reuptake inhibitor.

transitory neonatal respiratory and neurological distress after fluoxetine use throughout pregnancy (4), a prospective study did not suggest postnatal complications following in utero exposure to fluoxetine (5).

Another nonrandomized study (6) has suggested that third-trimester use of fluoxetine may increase the risk of perinatal complications and that first-trimester use of fluoxetine may increase the risk of unspecified "minor congenital anomalies." Nevertheless, because the control group in the study did not exclude depression as a confounding factor and because several other factors (e.g., maternal age) were uncontrolled, these results are difficult to interpret.

At the time of writing, no studies have assessed in utero exposure to the SSRIs sertraline, paroxetine, or fluvoxamine or to bupropion, trazodone, venlafaxine, or nefazodone.

Monoamine oxidase inhibitors (MAOIs) should be avoided in pregnancy, because they may produce a hypertensive crisis should tocolytic medications such as terbutaline be used to forestall premature labor. In addition, MAOIs have been associated in animal studies with an increased rate of congenital anomalies.

With regard to long-term neurobehavioral sequelae in children exposed in utero to antidepressants, reassuring results have recently been reported by researchers who followed the children of women who had received either tricyclic antidepressants or fluoxetine during pregnancy and compared the neurobehavioral development of these children to that of children of mothers who had not been exposed during pregnancy to any known teratogen (7). Results indicated that there were no significant differences in global IQ, temperament, mood, activity levels, distractibility, or behavior in any of the children, who were assessed between 16 and 86 months. Therefore, the use of fluoxetine when deemed to be required for the health and well-being of a pregnant woman and her fetus is probably safer than allowing a pregnant woman with severe, disabling depression to go untreated.

Mood Stabilizers

First-trimester use of lithium is associated with a 10- to 20-fold higher incidence of Ebstein's anomaly, a serious cardiac defect in which the tricuspid valve is displaced into the right ventricle (8, 9). Thus, although the risk of this anomaly is 1/20,000 in the general population, first-trimester exposure to lithium increases the risk up to 1/1000 (2, 10). Lithium use in pregnancy has been associated with neonatal symptoms including hypotonia, poor suck reflex, hypoglycemia, and cyanosis (11–13). Isolated cases of neonatal goiter and diabetes insipidus have also been reported (13). A 5-year follow-up study of children exposed to lithium in utero, based on questionnaires completed by the children's mothers, identified no neurobehavioral sequelae (14).

The data on the effects on the fetus of in utero anticonvulsants are limited, because most reports involve mothers who were treated for epilepsy, which itself is linked to an increased incidence of congenital malformations. After controlling for the increased risk of congenital malformations due to epilepsy, there nevertheless remains an increased risk for congenital anomalies in babies born to women treated with valproic acid and carbamazepine (2, 15). First-trimester exposure to valproic acid is associated with at least a 15-fold increase in the risk of spina bifida (elevating the risk from 6/10,000 to 90/10,000) and with facial abnormalities. Carbamazepine incurs a 1% risk of neural tube defects, including spina bifida. Developmental delay, craniofacial defects, and fingernail hypoplasia have been noted with both carbamazepine and valproic acid.

Antipsychotic Agents

Children born to unmedicated mothers with psychosis during pregnancy appear to have a twofold greater incidence of congenital anomalies (15). This increased risk may be due to genetic or other factors, e.g., inadequate prenatal care or substance abuse. The low-potency phenothiazines appear to increase the risk of nonspecific congenital anomalies, whereas high-potency neuroleptics—for example, haloperidol and trifluoperazine—are not associated with a greater rate of fetal anomalies (2). These data are largely based on the use of these medications for nausea and hyperemesis gravidarum, in which neuroleptics are used at low doses for their antiemetic effects. A single case report (16) of clozapine use in pregnancy showed no adverse effects. There are no data on risperidone use during pregnancy.

A transient perinatal syndrome of motor restlessness, tremor, hypotonia, hyperreflexia, irritability, dyskinesia, and poor feeding was reported in infants exposed to neuroleptics near term (2), and neonatal jaundice was reported with phenothiazines (17). Although in animals the use of neuroleptics appears to cause behavioral abnormalities, no neurobehavioral sequelae were noted in a single follow-up study in humans (18).

Agents to Treat Neuroleptic-Induced Extrapyramidal Side Effects

Prenatal exposure to the anticholinergic agents trihexyphenidyl and benztropine has been linked to minor congenital malformations, functional bowel obstruction, and urinary retention. Most studies suggest that diphenhydramine does not increase the risk of organ malformation; the drug may, however, produce perinatal withdrawal symptoms. Cardiovascular malformations have been noted with exposure to amantadine in utero (2).

Benzodiazepines

Data on the use of benzodiazepines in pregnancy are mixed: a significant risk of oral clefts has been noted in children born to women who took benzodiazepines in the first trimester (15). This risk has been noted particularly for diazepam and alprazolam. Data are also mixed on the risk of developmental delay in children exposed in utero to benzodiazepines. Exposure to these medications near delivery may cause decreased neonatal tone, failure to feed, temperature dysregulation, apnea, and low Apgar scores. Infrequent use of benzodiazepines during pregnancy, however, does not seem to be associated with neonatal difficulties.

Electroconvulsive Therapy

When carried out with a comprehensive treatment team consisting of a psychiatrist, anesthesiologist, and obstetrician, ECT appears to be a safe and effective treatment modality during pregnancy (2,19). It is the treatment of choice when rapid stabilization is essential (e.g., delusional depression, uncontrollable mania).

Preparation should include a pelvic examination, uterine tocodynamometry to rule out uterine contractions, and administration of a nonparticulate antacid such as sodium citrate to reduce the risk of gastric regurgitation, pulmonary aspiration, and aspiration pneumonitis. The patient should be hydrated and adequately oxygenated. During the ECT procedure, for patients in the later stages of pregnancy, the right hip should be elevated to maintain placental perfusion. Succinylcholine, a muscle relaxant frequently used during ECT, appears safe during pregnancy. During the procedure, an anticholinergic agent is used to prevent vagal bradycardia and to decrease throat and tracheal secretions. Atropine, sometimes used to prevent vagal bradycardia and decrease respiratory and gastrointestinal secretions, is contraindicated in pregnancy because it rapidly passes across the placenta, causes fetal tachycardia and variable heart rate, and may mask signs of fetal distress. The anticholinergic agent glycopyrrolate is much less likely to cross the placenta and is therefore a safer alternative. Short-acting barbiturates do not appear to affect the fetus adversely (19).

External fetal monitoring should continue for several hours after ECT (Table 4–6).

■ COURSE AND MANAGEMENT OF PSYCHIATRIC DISORDERS DURING PREGNANCY

Depression

The incidence of depression (both major and minor) in pregnancy is approximately 10%, comparable to that in nonpregnant women. Risk factors for depression in pregnancy include younger age, lack of social support, living alone, and having more children (15). Depression during pregnancy triples the risk for postpartum depression and is linked to inadequate prenatal care, poor nutrition, and suicide (20). Depressed pregnant women may be at risk for preterm deliveries and babies small for their gestational age (21).

As for all psychotropic agents during pregnancy, antidepressants should be reserved for use only when the risk of not

---

TABLE 4–6. **Electroconvulsive therapy (ECT) for the pregnant patient**

Before ECT

    Perform pelvic examination

    Perform uterine tocodynamometry

    Give antacid: sodium citrate

    Begin adequate hydration, continue during procedure

During ECT

    Oxygenate

    Elevate right hip

    Administer succinylcholine for muscle relaxation

    Administer anticholinergic glycopyrrolate

---

treating an illness in the mother outweighs the possible risk of treatment (Table 4–7). When depressive symptoms are mild or moderate, nonpharmacological interventions should be undertaken, particularly in the first trimester. They include psychotherapy, conjoint counseling, modalities to reduce stress, and mobilization of available environmental psychosocial supports. When symptoms are severe (i.e., the patient is suicidal, psychotic, or not gaining weight), the risk of treatment with medication may be outweighed by the risk of nontreatment. Current data have shown that TCAs and fluoxetine are relatively safe during pregnancy (2). Of the TCAs, it is best to choose either nortriptyline or desipramine, because they produce fewer anticholinergic and hypotensive effects than other TCAs and because blood levels may be followed during pregnancy. Blood levels of medication may drop as pregnancy progresses, possibly because of increased hepatic metabolism and/or greater volume of distribution. It may therefore be necessary to increase antidepressant doses in order to achieve pregravid therapeutic blood levels (22). Fluoxetine is a reasonable option, although until more data exist on its use during pregnancy, it should be reserved for patients who have been refractory to

---

TABLE 4–7. **Risks associated with psychiatric disorders during pregnancy**

Poor prenatal care

Malnutrition

Fetal abuse or neonaticide

Failure to recognize or report signs of labor

Suicide

Poor pregnancy outcomes: low birth weight, preterm delivery; lower Apgar scores

Impulsive behavior (reckless driving, promiscuity)

Use of street drugs, alcohol

TCAs. It is best to avoid the use of the other SSRIs or the newer antidepressants until more is learned about their safety in pregnancy. Hospitalization and/or ECT should be considered for a suicidal or delusionally depressed pregnant woman.

Bipolar Disorder

Little is known about the course of bipolar disorder across pregnancy. Hospital admissions for bipolar illness appear to drop during pregnancy, compared to non–pregnancy-related admissions (23), but it may be that increased contact with health practitioners through prenatal visits helps protect against relapse.

All three mood stabilizers commonly used to treat bipolar disorder (lithium, carbamazepine, and valproic acid) are associated with increased rates of fetal anomalies when used in the first trimester. Thus, for women with long periods of interepisode well-being, it is worth trying to discontinue these medications prior to conception. Medications should be tapered gradually (i.e., over a 4-week period), because abrupt medication discontinuation increases the risk of relapse (24).

When possible, mood stabilizers should be avoided during the first trimester of pregnancy. However, for women with a history of decompensation when not on medication, pharmacotherapy may need to be continued during pregnancy. A relapse of mania poses grave dangers to both a mother and the fetus: poor judgment and impulsive behavior may result in reckless driving, drug abuse, and failure to obtain prenatal care. Dysphoric and psychotic manic episodes are even more hazardous, for they place the patient at risk of suicide and fetal abuse. Because of the more teratogenic potential of carbamazepine and valproic acid, lithium is the mood stabilizer of choice in pregnancy. It should be prescribed in multiple daily dosing to avoid exposing the fetus to peak blood levels. Lithium levels should be followed at least monthly, because they may drop with the increase in maternal fluid volume and in renal clearance. A level II ultrasound should be obtained at week 18 to assess for cardiovascular anomalies. Approximately 2 weeks before the estimated date of delivery, the lithium dose should be tapered by approximately one-third to one-half to avoid lithium toxicity in the mother following the rapid fluid shifts occurring after delivery.

ECT is an alternative treatment for women who experience an exacerbation or escalation of symptoms despite other treatment interventions. In cases when carbamazepine or valproic acid cannot be discontinued in the first trimester, an amniotic α-fetoprotein analysis at gestational week 16 and an ultrasound during weeks 18–22 can screen for neural tube defects. Folate supplementation may reduce the incidence of neural tube defects and should be provided for all women 4 weeks before conception is attempted and through the first trimester (2).

Schizophrenia

Schizophrenia has a variable course during pregnancy: some women experience improvement, whereas others deteriorate (25). Older maternal age and fewer physical complications are predictive of better course (26). Regardless of the course, schizophrenic women require close follow-up during pregnancy. A relapse or exacerbation of psychosis requires aggressive interventions. Psychosis in pregnancy can lead to fetal abuse or neonaticide, failure to obtain prenatal care, inability to care for oneself, and inability to recognize or report signs of labor. A reduction of psychotic symptoms during pregnancy decreases the likelihood of adverse pregnancy outcomes (prematurity, low birth weight, low Apgar scores) (15). Important interventions include assessment for substance abuse, reduction of psychosocial stressors, and mobilization of family support. Close collaboration with the obstetrical team facilitates the patient's cooperation with necessary medical procedures.

Chronically mentally ill women have a high incidence of

losing their children to foster care or adoption. When it appears that the patient may be unable to provide adequate parenting, social service assistance should be requested. Steps can be taken to teach parenting skills, to set up adequate housing, to mobilize family support, and to organize financial assistance (Table 4–8).

When possible, neuroleptics should be avoided during the first trimester. For pregnant patients in whom neuroleptic use is deemed necessary (e.g., patients experiencing command hallucinations to harm themselves or the fetus; patients unable to care for themselves appropriately because of paranoia or thought disorganization), neuroleptic use as needed may be preferable to regular daily use during the first trimester. However, for refractory and severely disabled psychotic patients, daily dosing may be necessary. For women requiring antipsychotic medication during pregnancy, it is advisable to use high-potency neuroleptics such as haloperidol or trifluoperazine, because data on their use in pregnancy appear more favorable than for low-potency medications and because the high-potency medications are less likely to produce anticholinergic and hypotensive side effects. Doses should be maintained at the minimum necessary for symptom control. Most agents to treat extrapyramidal side effects are best avoided in pregnancy, because they are associated with major and minor congenital anomalies; most studies suggest that diphenhydramine does not increase the risk of congenital malformation. Alternative

---

TABLE 4–8. **Important factors to assess in the chronically mentally ill pregnant patient**

Social service needs

Custody issues

Parenting skills

Need for financial assistance

strategies for patients who experience extrapyramidal symptoms include reduction of the neuroleptic dose and switching to a lower-potency agent.

A pregnant psychotic woman who refuses prenatal care presents complicated ethical and legal issues. Often the patient can be engaged in treatment through education and support. If the patient's psychosis interferes with her capacity to make informed decisions about her treatment, her psychiatric condition should be treated. If she refuses psychiatric care or is unable to make an informed decision despite the psychiatric care, a court order may be necessary in order to proceed with obstetrical interventions. Psychiatric care can also be enforced if the patient is deemed to be a danger to herself or to others or to be gravely disabled. Whether a pregnant woman who engages in behaviors that are potentially harmful to the fetus can be considered a "danger to others" is a matter of significant legal controversy.

Anxiety Disorders

Little is known about the course of generalized anxiety disorder during pregnancy. The symptoms of panic disorder improve in some women and worsen in others. Obsessive-compulsive disorder (OCD) appears to worsen during pregnancy (27).

Factors contributing to the course of anxiety disorders in pregnancy include concerns about one's changing roles and responsibilities and the impact of a new child on one's professional, social, and family life. Increased heart rate and minute ventilation may also contribute to anxiety, because it has been speculated that panic attacks result from catastrophic cognitive reactions to normal physiological events (28). On the other hand, progesterone and its metabolites, both very high in pregnancy, are active at the γ-aminobutyric acid (GABA) receptor and have sedating qualities that may help protect against anxiety attacks.

Cognitive-behavior therapy is an effective treatment for many patients with panic disorder and OCD, and it should be considered as an alternative to medication. Additional non-pharmacological interventions include elimination of caffeine and nicotine, reduction of psychosocial stressors, and family or couple therapy.

When symptoms are severe and require more aggressive intervention, the TCAs and fluoxetine are reasonable treatment options. Benzodiazepines may be necessary initially until the antidepressant medications take effect. Benzodiazepines should be used at the lowest possible dosage and if possible avoided during the period of oral cleft closure (weeks 6–9). Intermittent use of small doses of benzodiazepines may be necessary at various points during pregnancy. Lorazepam is a reasonable choice because it has no active metabolites and appears to cross into the placenta at a lower rate than do other benzodiazepines (29). Clonazepam is an alternative for patients who require a longer-acting sedative effect. To reduce the risk of toxicity and withdrawal symptoms in the neonate, the use of benzodiazepines should be kept at a minimum near term. To avoid in utero withdrawal, benzodiazepines should be tapered rather than discontinued abruptly during pregnancy. No human data exist for the anxiolytic agent buspirone in pregnancy.

Eating Disorders

For many bulimic and anorexic women, the weight gain of pregnancy represents a failure of the effort to maintain a certain weight and may therefore be difficult to tolerate. Eating disorders during pregnancy increase the risk for complications, including pregnancy-induced hypertension and depression, intrauterine growth retardation, congenital malformations, and failure to thrive (30).

Patients with eating disorders should be encouraged to

avoid conception until their symptoms have abated. Psycho-therapy before and during the pregnancy is important to help reduce the distress these patients may experience from their changing body shape. Cognitive-behavior therapy is a particularly effective treatment strategy for bulimia nervosa. When the eating disorder poses a risk to the woman and/or fetus (electrolyte imbalance from vomiting, malnutrition, inadequate weight gain), pharmacotherapy may be necessary. TCAs and fluoxetine are helpful, particularly for bulimia. It is of note that women with anorexia nervosa have a high incidence of amenorrhea and may have difficulty conceiving.

■ SUBSTANCE ABUSE AND PREGNANCY

Rates of alcohol and substance abuse in women have been rising in the past decade, particularly for cocaine (31). Recent figures show that approximately 5%–6% of adult American women meet criteria for alcohol or substance abuse and/or dependence (32). Particularly at risk are women of reproductive age (33). Alcohol and illicit drugs are of great concern during pregnancy, because they are associated with an increased incidence of negative obstetrical and perinatal outcomes (Table 4–9).

Tobacco

Although tobacco is not an illegal drug, its use during pregnancy increases the risk of obstetrical complications and perinatal morbidity. Tobacco has been implicated in spontaneous abortion, placenta praevia, and abruptio placentae (32). Cigarette smoking has been linked to intrauterine growth retardation, low birth weight, and preterm delivery. The deficits associated with in utero exposure to tobacco do not appear to be overcome by age 3 and may include sustained cognitive deficits (31).

TABLE 4–9. Commonly reported teratogenic effects of abused drugs

Specific fetal effects	Opiates	Alcohol	Other sedative-hypnotic drugs	Cocaine	Other stimulants	Halluci-nogens	Marijuana	Nicotine
Structural nonspecific growth retardation	X	X	-	X	-	-	X	X
Specific dysmorphic effects	-	X	-	X	-	-	-	-
Behavioral	X	X	X	X	X	X	X	X
Neurobiochemical (abstinence syndrome)	X	X	X	-	-	-	-	-
Increased fetal and perinatal mortality	X	X	-	X	-	-	-	-
Percentage of women reporting use in pregnancy (varies with population)	5	> 50	< 5	≤ 20	< 5	< 5	5–34	> 50

Note. – = effect not reported.
Source. Reprinted from Hoegerman G, Wilson CA, Thurmond E, et al.: "Drug-Exposed Neonates." *Western Journal of Medicine* 152:559–564, 1990. Used with permission.

Alcohol

Although the negative effect of alcohol on pregnancy and the developing fetus is due to a combination of pharmacological, lifestyle, and nutritional factors, it is clear that alcohol has direct adverse effects on obstetrical course and on the developing fetus. Alcohol displaces proteins, vitamins, and essential fats needed for proper fetal development and, with its metabolite, acetaldehyde, is directly toxic to fetal cellular growth and metabolism. Alcohol's teratogenic effects produce a spectrum of congenital anomalies ranging from the *fetal alcohol syndrome* to isolated abnormalities termed *fetal alcohol effects* (31) (Tables 4–10 and 4–11). The incidence of fetal alcohol syndrome is 1–2 live births per 1,000, and fetal alcohol effects occur at an estimated rate of 3–5 live births per 1,000. In utero daily exposure to 89 mL or more of alcohol (about three

TABLE 4–10. **Principal features of fetal alcohol syndrome**

Structural
　Shortened palpebral fissures
　Hypoplastic philtrum and maxilla
　Thinned upper vermilion border
　Retrognathia in infancy
　Micrognathia/prognathia in adolescence
　Diminished adipose tissue
Cognitive
　Mild to moderate mental retardation
Behavioral
　Poor coordination, hypotonia
　Irritability in infancy
　Attention deficit with hyperactivity in childhood
Growth retardation
　Height and weight below 95th percentile

Source.　Adapted from McCance-Katz 1991 (31). Used with permission.

TABLE 4–11.	**Principal features of fetal alcohol effects**

Ptosis, strabismus, epicanthal folds

Posterior rotation of ears

Prominent lateral palatine ridges

Cardiac murmurs, atrial septal defects

Labial hypoplasia

Hemangiomas

Abnormal palmar creases, pectus excavatum

Source. Reprinted from McCance-Katz EF: "The Consequences of Maternal Substance Abuse for the Child Exposed in Utero." *Psychosomatics* 32:268–274, 1991. Used with permission.

1-ounce drinks of hard liquor) is associated with a serious risk of fetal alcohol syndrome. Nevertheless, no safe level of alcohol consumption has been established. Women should be encouraged to abstain from alcohol during pregnancy, because it is possible that even occasional consumption may result in fetal defects (31).

In addition to its teratogenic effects, alcohol has been associated with premature labor, abruptio placentae, stillbirth, and other obstetrical complications. Alcohol may also suppress uterine contractions, thus prolonging labor.

Cocaine

Adverse effects on the fetus of cocaine use in pregnancy result in part from its acute toxic effects on the mother. Cocaine produces maternal hypertension and tachycardia, with subsequent reduction of placental blood flow, placental vasoconstriction, and reduced oxygen transport to the fetus. Cocaine may also have teratogenic potential: babies exposed to in utero cocaine appear to be at risk for genitourinary tract malformations (31).

Cocaine's vasoconstrictive effect and its tendency to cause cardiac arrhythmias increase the risk for obstetrical complications, including preterm labor and abruptio placentae. Intrauterine growth retardation is increased, and fetal distress during labor may occur; neonates may have lower Apgar scores and fetal meconium staining.

A prolonged abstinence syndrome, lasting up to 4 months, also occurs in neonates exposed to in utero cocaine. The syndrome is characterized by tremulousness, lability of mood, abnormal motor development, persistence of primitive reflexes, and impaired bonding. Extended behavioral abnormalities in babies born to cocaine-abusing mothers include mood dysfunction and decreased ability to experience pleasure.

Opiates

Heroin use during pregnancy has been associated with an increased incidence of obstetrical complications, including intrauterine growth retardation, premature rupture of membranes, pregnancy-induced hypertension (toxemia of pregnancy), abruptio placentae, neonatal meconium aspiration, maternal and neonatal infections, and stillbirth.

A perinatal withdrawal syndrome has also been reported, including irritability, decreased feeding, respiratory difficulties, sweating, and tremulousness. This syndrome may be minimized by the use of low-dose methadone and appropriate perinatal care. Women maintained on methadone who receive proper prenatal care have improved obstetrical outcome compared with women with untreated opiate use (32).

Other adverse effects associated with in utero exposure to opiates include low birth weight, decreased head circumference, and increased risk of sudden infant death syndrome (SIDS).

Cannabis (Marijuana)

Cannabis is fat soluble and therefore crosses the placenta readily. Once cannabis is in the fetal circulation, its excretion is delayed, and full clearance may not occur for up to 30 days following exposure. Cannabis elevates carbon monoxide levels in the mother and thus decreases fetal oxygenation. Fetal hypoxia also occurs from cannabis-induced maternal tachycardia and hypertension, which reduce placental blood flow.

Treatment

Goals of the treatment of pregnant substance- and alcohol-abusing women include eliminating alcohol and drug use, treating comorbid medical or psychiatric disorders, assisting the patient safely through the pregnancy, providing assistance for training in parenting skills, and facilitating the patient's continued treatment after pregnancy (34).

The most important approach to managing the chemically dependent pregnant patient is to provide treatment options in a nonjudgmental and empathic therapeutic setting. Although it is useful to provide the patient with information regarding the harmful effects of alcohol and drugs on obstetrical and fetal outcome, the information should be delivered in the context of managing the substance abuse. Emphasis should be placed on working on a plan to achieve abstinence in order to maximize a return to health for both the mother and the developing baby.

Although pregnancy offers a window of opportunity for treating substance abuse, patients who abuse substances often relapse after pregnancy (at a time when they are responsible for the care of their infant). Rehabilitation, detoxification, and ongoing supportive treatment are necessary in order to treat the patient during pregnancy and to maximize the opportunity for prolonged success following delivery. A multidimensional approach to treating these patients is essential. The treatment team should include infant and child health care providers, mental health care providers, social service workers, and substance abuse counselors. Attention to practical needs, such as the provision of transportation and child care services, facilitates compliance with a coordinated treatment approach.

Opiate-dependent pregnant women may be detoxified or switched to a methadone maintenance program. Self-help fellowships (Alcoholics Anonymous, Narcotics Anonymous, and Women for Sobriety) are useful. To optimize support for the patient during and after the pregnancy, family members or significant others should be involved. They may benefit from referrals to self-help programs (Al-Anon and Nar-Anon) and to mental health counseling.

The obstetrician and pediatrician should be informed about the nature of the substance use, abuse, or dependence, and all professionals should work closely to support the patient medically, psychiatrically, and obstetrically and to ensure the good care of the infant following delivery.

■ REFERENCES

1. Key to FDA use-in-pregnancy ratings, in Physicians' Desk Reference, 50th Edition. Montvale, NJ, Medical Economics Data Production, 1996, unnumbered page (11th from end of volume)
2. Altshuler L, Cohen L, Szuba MP, et al: Pharmacologic management of psychiatric illness in pregnancy: dilemmas and guidelines. Am J Psychiatry 153:592–606, 1996
3. Pastuszak A, Schick-Boschetto B, Zuber C, et al: Pregnancy outcome following first-trimester exposure to fluoxetine (Prozac). JAMA 269:2246–2248, 1993
4. Spencer MJ: Fluoxetine hydrochloride (Prozac) toxicity in a neonate. Pediatrics 92:721–722, 1993
5. Goldstein DJ: Effects of third trimester fluoxetine exposure on the newborn. J Clin Psychopharmacol 15:417–420, 1995
6. Chambers CD, Johnson KA, Dick BA, et al: Birth outcomes in pregnant women taking fluoxerine. N Engl J Med 335:1010–1015, 1996
7. Nulman I, Rovet J, Stewart DE, et al: Neurodevelopment of children exposed in utero to antidepressant drugs. N Engl J Med 336:258–262, 1997
8. Schou M, Goldfield MD, Weinstein MR, et al: Lithium and preg-

nancy, I: report from the register of lithium babies. Br Med J 2:135–136, 1973

9. Weinstein MR, Goldfield MD: Cardiovascular malformations with lithium use during pregnancy. Am J Psychiatry 132:529–531, 1975

10. Cohen LS, Friedman JM, Jefferson JW, et al: A re-evaluation of risk of in utero exposure to lithium. JAMA 271:146–150, 1994

11. Schou M, Amdisen A: Lithium and the placenta (letter). Am J Obstet Gynecol 122:541, 1975

12. Woody JN, London WL, Wilbanks GD: Lithium toxicity in a newborn. Pediatrics 47:94–86, 1971

13. Miller LJ: Psychiatric medication during pregnancy: understanding and minimizing risks. Psychiatric Annals 24:69–75, 1994

14. Schou ML: What happened to the lithium babies: a followup study of children born without malformations. Acta Psychiatr Scand 54:193–197, 1976

15. Altshuler LL, Hendrick V, Cohen L, et al: The use of psychotropics in the pregnant patient, in Current Psychiatric Therapy II. Edited by Dunner D. Philadelphia, PA, WB Saunders, in press

16. Waldman M, Safferman A: Pregnancy and clozapine (letter). Am J Psychiatr 150:168–169, 1993

17. Scokel PW, Jones WD: Infant jaundice after phenothiazine drugs for labor: an enigma. Obstet Gynecol 20:124–127, 1962

18. Slone D, Siskind V, Heinomen OP, et al: Antenatal exposure to the phenothiazines in relation to congenital malformations, perinatal mortality rate, birth weight and intelligence quotient score. Am J Obstet Gynecol 128:486–488, 1977

19. Miller LJ: Use of electroconvulsive therapy during pregnancy. Hosp Commun Psychiatry 45:444–450, 1994

20. O'Hara MW: Summary and implications, in Postpartum Depression: Causes and Consequences. New York, Springer-Verlag, 1993, pp 168–194

21. Steer RA, Scholl TO, Hediger ML, et al: Self-reported depression and negative pregnancy outcomes. J Clin Epidemiol 45:1093–1099, 1992

22. Altshuler LL, Hendrick V: Pregnancy and psychotropic medication: changes in blood levels. J Clin Psychopharmacol 16:78–80, 1996

23. Kastrup M, Lier L, Rafaelsen OJ: Psychiatric illness in relation to pregnancy and childbirth, I: methodologic considerations. Nordisk

Psykiatrisk Tidsskrift 43:531–534, 1989

24. Faedda GL, Tondo L, Baldessariini RJ, et al: Outcome after rapid vs gradual discontinuation of lithium treatment in bipolar disorders. Arch Gen Psychiatry 50:448–455, 1993

25. McNeil TF, Kaij L, Malmquist-Larsson A: Women with nonorganic psychosis: pregnancy's effect on mental health during pregnancy. Acta Psychiatr Scand 70:140–148, 1984

26. McNeil TF, Kaij L, Malmquist-Larsson A: Women with nonorganic psychosis: factors associated with pregnancy's effect on mental health. Acta Psychiatr Scand 70:209–219, 1984

27. Buttolph ML, Holland DA: Obsessive-compulsive disorders in pregnancy and childbirth, in Obsessive Compulsive Disorders: Theory and Management. Edited by Jenike MA, Baier L, Minichiello WE. Chicago, IL, Year Book Medical, 1990, pp 89–95

28. Cowley DS, Roy-Byrne RP: Panic disorder during pregnancy. J Psychosom Obstet Gynaecol 10:193–210, 1989

29. Whitelaw AGL, Cummings AJ, McFadyen IR: Effect of maternal lorazepam on the neonate. BMJ 282:1106–1108, 1981

30. Lacey JH, Smith G: Bulimia nervosa: the impact of pregnancy on mother and baby. Br J Psychiatry 150:777–781, 1987

31. McCance-Katz EF: The consequences of maternal substance abuse for the child exposed in utero. Psychosomatics 32:268–274, 1991

32. Blume SB, Russell M: Alcohol and substance abuse in the practice of obstetrics and gynecology, in Psychological Aspects of Women's Health Care: The Interface Between Psychiatry and Obstetrics and Gynecology. Edited by Stewart DE, Stotland NL. Washington, DC, American Psychiatric Press, pp 391–409, 1993

33. Silverman S: Scope, specifics of maternal drug use, effect on fetus are beginning to emerge from studies. JAMA 261:117–129, 1986

34. Work Group on Substance Use Disorders: Practice guidelines for the treatment of patients with substance use disorders: alcohol, cocaine, opioids. Am J Psychiatry 152 (suppl 11):26, 1995

POSTPARTUM PSYCHIATRIC DISORDERS

For many women, the months following delivery are a time of vulnerability for psychiatric disorders. The incidence of psychiatric admissions increases significantly in the first 6 months postpartum compared to other times in a woman's life (1) (Figure 5–1). Postpartum mood syndromes are generally classified as postpartum blues *(maternity blues),* postpartum depression, and postpartum psychosis (Table 5–1). Whether these three disorders represent distinct syndromes or rather a continuum is unclear. It is known, however, that these disorders can disrupt family life, have a negative effect on the development of the infant, and increase the risk of subsequent psychopathology in the mother.

■ POSTPARTUM BLUES

The mildest and most common of the postpartum syndromes is postpartum blues (maternity blues), a transitory state beginning within the first 2–4 days after delivery and lasting no more than 2 weeks. Typical symptoms include tearfulness, mood lability, irritability, and anxiety. The condition occurs in up to 85% of all new mothers (2) and is thus an expected transient reaction following delivery. Women and their partners benefit from support and reassurance that their symptoms are com-

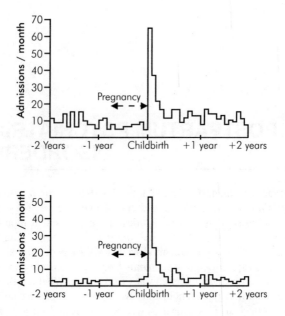

FIGURE 5–1. **Hospital admissions in the 2 years preceding and following delivery.** *Top,* all admissions. *Bottom,* psychosis admissions. *Source.* Reprinted from Kendell RE, Chalmers JC, Platz C: p. 664 in "Epidemiology of puerperal psychoses." *Br J Psychiatry* 150:662–673, 1987. Used with permission.

mon and will end soon. Because new mothers are frequently discharged from the hospital on the first or second postpartum day, it may be helpful to provide some information regarding this condition to women prior to delivery.

Risk Factors

A history of depression, particularly depression during pregnancy, increases the risk of postpartum blues. A history

TABLE 5-1. Postpartum disorders: incidence, time course, and clinical features

Disorder	Incidence (%)	Time course	Clinical features
Postpartum blues	70–85	Onset within first postpartum week, abates after 10–14 days	Mood instability, tearfulness, anxiety, insomnia
Postpartum depression	10	Onset within first postpartum month; duration similar to that of major depressive episode	Depressed mood, guilt, anxiety, fear of harm coming to baby, obsessional features
Postpartum psychosis	0.1–0.2	Onset within first postpartum month; duration variable—weeks to months	Disorientation, confusion. delusions, hallucinations, often rapid mood cycling

of premenstrual dysphoric disorder also appears to be a risk factor.

Treatment

Because postpartum blues are transitory and have no long-term consequences, medical and psychiatric interventions are not necessary. Reassurance, support, and education are enough in most cases. Women should be monitored to ensure that their symptoms do not persist or grow into a postpartum depression.

■ POSTPARTUM DEPRESSION

Postpartum depression tends to have a later onset than postpartum blues, beginning usually at 2–4 weeks postpartum. Recent prevalence data suggest a 10% risk of major depression in the postpartum period, a rate equaling that in the general female population (3). Nevertheless, postpartum women do appear to have increased rates of depressive symptomatology (3). Depressive symptoms occurring during the postpartum period deserve special attention because they cause considerable distress for the patient and her family. The potential negative consequences of postpartum depression to the emotional and cognitive development of the infant add to the importance of diagnosing and treating this condition (2). Failure to diagnose postpartum depression may arise in part from the focus on the well-being of the baby rather than that of the mother following delivery. New mothers, sensing societal expectations that they be content and fulfilled, may be reluctant to reveal their feelings. Furthermore, families and physicians may dismiss a woman's symptoms, attributing them solely to the stress of looking after a newborn child.

Risk Factors

A history of nonpuerperal depression is associated with a 24% risk of postpartum depression (3). Depression occurring during pregnancy is associated with a still higher risk, 35% (3). A previous postpartum depression is a particularly significant risk factor for recurrence, conferring a recurrence risk of up to 50% (4). Stressful life events and a lack of support, particularly from the woman's spouse or partner, also increase the risk of postpartum depression (Table 5–2). Socioeconomic factors, age, obstetrical complications, and breast-feeding do not appear to be associated with postpartum depression (3).

Treatment

The most successful treatment strategies are multifactorial. They include education, psychotherapy, group support, referrals to self-help and national organizations (Table 5–3), and conjoint counseling if the relationship with the partner is problematic.

TABLE 5–2. **Risk factors for postpartum disorders**

Disorder	Risk factors
Postpartum blues	Depressive symptoms during pregnancy
	History of depression
	History of premenstrual dysphoric disorder
Postpartum depression	Depression during pregnancy
	History of depression, especially postpartum depression
	Dysfunctional marital relationship
	Inadequate social supports
	Stressful life events during pregnancy
Postpartum psychosis	History of bipolar disorder
	Primiparity
	Previous postpartum psychosis

TABLE 5–3. **Treatment options for postpartum disorders**

Disorder	Treatment options
Postpartum blues	Education
	Support
	Reassurance
Postpartum depression	Mobilization of family supports: partner, other family members
	Reduction of psychosocial stressors
	Individual and/or group psychotherapy
	Antidepressant medications
	Electroconvulsive therapy (ECT)
	Hospitalization
Postpartum psychosis	Hospitalization
	Medical workup to rule out organic etiology
	Mood stabilizers
	Neuroleptics
	Antidepressants
	Benzodiazepines
	ECT

The patient should be encouraged to obtain support from family and friends for infant care, to get as much sleep and rest as possible, and to reduce her other responsibilities. If possible, hiring a child care assistant for even part of each day is extremely helpful. Standard antidepressant medications are often very effective. For women with a history of postpartum depression, antidepressants begun at the time of delivery may significantly protect against a relapse (5). The decision to use medications should take into consideration whether the patient will be breast-feeding. Spouses and partners should be involved in the treatment, because their support is essential for successful management of the postpartum depression.

■ POSTPARTUM PSYCHOSIS

Postpartum psychosis is an acute, severe illness occurring in 1–2 of every 1,000 births (2). Symptoms include lability of mood, severe agitation, confusion, thought disorganization, hallucinations, and sleeplessness. Many researchers believe that postpartum psychosis is a manifestation of bipolar disorder. Following an episode of postpartum psychosis, women are at risk of subsequent nonpostpartum manic-depressive relapses (6).

Risk Factors

A significant risk factor for postpartum psychosis is a history of manic-depressive illness, which confers a risk of approximately 35% (1). A previous postpartum psychosis is associated with a 20%–33% risk of relapse following a subsequent delivery (1, 7, 8). Women with a history of both bipolar disorder and postpartum psychosis have a 50% chance of recurrence of postpartum psychosis following subsequent deliveries (8). Primiparity and a family history of bipolar disorder also increase the risk (2). A diagnosis of schizophrenia does not appear to be a significant risk factor (1).

Treatment

Because patients with postpartum psychosis are at risk for child neglect, child abuse, infanticide, and suicide, psychiatric hospitalization is almost always indicated. A medical workup to rule out organic etiologies (e.g., postpartum thyroiditis, Sheehan's syndrome, human immunodeficiency virus [HIV] infection, intoxication/withdrawal states, pregnancy-related autoimmune disorders, an intracranial mass) should be undertaken. Mood stabilizers should be initiated immediately, and neuroleptics are often necessary for acute psychosis and agitation. Although antidepressants are beneficial for patients with depressive psychosis, they should be used with caution in postpartum psychosis, because there is a risk of precipitating a protracted and complicated course with rapid mood cycling (9). Electroconvulsive therapy is an important treatment alternative for patients who do not respond to pharmacotherapy or whose symptoms appear to be escalating.

Patients with a single episode of psychosis occurring in the postpartum period appear to have a better long-term course than do patients with psychotic illnesses occurring at other times of their lives (6). Nevertheless, the risk of subsequent affective episodes is relatively high. Following an initial psychotic illness in the postpartum period, the probability of a recurrent affective illness has been reported at approximately 60% (7, 10).

Thus, a patient with a postpartum psychosis is at risk for nonpuerperal relapses. For a patient with a history of affective illness, maintenance treatment with a mood stabilizer is indicated. If there is no history of affective or psychotic episodes and if the patient prefers not to keep taking medication, mood stabilizers and/or neuroleptics can be tapered and discontinued at 9–12 months postpartum. She should be warned, however, of her risk of relapse and of warning signs of recurrent illness. If she becomes pregnant again, mood stabilizers should be used prophylactically, beginning in the third trimester or at delivery. Although the proportion of first-episode postpartum psychoses that are eventually diagnosed as schizophrenic appears low (10), women with schizophreniform symptoms in the postpartum period have a poorer course (7, 10) and may require maintenance treatment with a neuroleptic. Time of onset of symptoms influences the long-term prognosis: new-onset psychosis that develops within 3 weeks of delivery appears to have a more favorable course than a psychosis developing later in the postpartum period.

Patients with a history of bipolar disorder are at significant risk for postpartum psychosis. For these patients, initiation of a mood stabilizer either in the third trimester or immediately after delivery can significantly reduce the rate of relapse (11).

■ ETIOLOGY OF POSTPARTUM MOOD DISORDERS

The etiology of postpartum disorders is unknown. A number of biological factors, including levels of estrogen, progesterone, cortisol, tryptophan, thyroid hormones, β-endorphin, and pro-lactin, have been speculated to play a role, but studies have been negative or contradictory (2). In animal models, estrogen has an antidopaminergic effect, similar to that of neuroleptics (12). Estrogen depletion appears to produce dopamine receptor supersensitivity and may predispose to psychosis (13).

Psychological factors probably play a role in postpartum depression. For example, the blues may reflect a letdown following the stress and excitement of pregnancy and childbirth (3). Psychological factors that may increase vulnerability to postpartum depressive symptoms include a low sense of self-control and maladaptive cognitions (3). Although incidence rates of postpartum psychosis appear consistent across cultures and ethnic groups (14), postpartum depression is reported to occur less frequently in some non-Western societies. In particular, rates of postpartum depression appear lower in cultures where women receive assistance, appreciation of their new roles as mothers, education about the techniques of mothering, and an opportunity to rest following the delivery (15).

It is unlikely that a single etiology accounts for postpartum mood disorders. Biological, social, and psychological factors probably contribute—to varying degrees in different women.

■ BREAST-FEEDING AND PSYCHOTROPIC MEDICATIONS

About half of new mothers breast-feed. Breast-feeding not only enhances maternal-infant bonding but also offers health benefits to the baby. Breast milk contains antibodies, enzymes, hormones, growth factors, and other compounds that foster maturation of the infant's digestive tract (16) and protect against pathogens. Respiratory and urinary tract infections occur less frequently in breast-fed than in bottle-fed infants. However, because little is known about the risks to an infant of exposure to medications through breast milk, clinicians and patients often choose to forgo breast-feeding. Fortunately, data on the use of psychotropic medication in breast-feeding women are increasingly reassuring, because more case reports note no adverse effects in lactating infants exposed to medication. Nevertheless, no medication should be used in a breast-feeding woman without a careful consideration of the risks and benefits. Other treatment approaches, including individual and group psychotherapy and reduction of psychosocial stressors, should be attempted before psychotropic agents are used. If these approaches fail, or if the woman chooses to use medication after being thoroughly informed of alternative treatments, a careful discussion with the woman and her partner should ensue. This discussion should review the available data on breast-feeding and psychotropic medication use, including what is known about risks and benefits. It is important that a pediatrician who is aware of the breast-feeding mother's use of medication monitor the infant for potential adverse sequelae.

■ GUIDELINES FOR USE OF PSYCHOTROPIC MEDICATIONS IN BREAST-FEEDING MOTHERS

To establish the infant's baseline of behavior, sleep and feeding patterns, and alertness, a pediatric assessment should be obtained before breast-feeding is begun. To minimize the infant's medication exposure, the mother should be prescribed the minimum dosage of medication that achieves remission of her psychiatric symptoms. If her symptoms do not improve with pharmacotherapy, a reevaluation of the risk-benefit discussion is warranted.

Other considerations in the use of psychotropic medications during breast-feeding include the use of short-acting rather than long-acting medications and supplementation with bottle feeding to reduce the infant's exposure to the drug. The measurement of breast milk levels of medication across a 24-hour period allows for determination of times in the day when breast milk concentrations peak and breast-feeding is thus best avoided.

Once the mother's medication serum levels are at steady state, the infant's serum should be assayed for levels of both the parent drug and its metabolites. Laboratories should be requested to use assays at the lowest limits of sensitivity. It is reassuring to find that the infant's levels are not detectable, although the clinical significance of detectable levels, even at the lower limits of detectability, is not known. Available data, however, show that adverse effects to infants are rarely associated with levels of 10 ng/mL or below.

Table 5–4 summarizes current knowledge, mostly derived from case reports, on the use of psychotropic medications in breast-feeding women. Most medications have been classified by the American Academy of Pediatrics (AAP) as "drugs whose effect on nursing infants is unknown but may be of concern" (31). These medications include the tricyclic antidepressants, the benzodiazepines, and the neuroleptics. Lithium, however, is contraindicated by the Academy's Committee on Drugs, because adverse effects have been noted in exposed infants. Although MAOIs are not included in the Academy's listing, they should not be used in breast-feeding because of the risk of hypertension in the infant. The Academy lists carbamazepine and valproic acid among drugs that "are usually compatible with breast-feeding" (31). However, because valproic acid exposure has been associated with hepatotoxicity in infants, it should be used with caution in breast-feeding women.

TABLE 5–4. Psychotropic drugs in breast-feeding

Medication	Comment	References
Tricyclic antidepressants (TCAs)	Considerable interindividual variability in breast milk levels and in ratios of breast milk to maternal plasma. With exception of single case of sedation and respiratory depression in an infant exposed to doxepin through breast milk, case reports do not show adverse effects in breast-fed infants exposed to TCAs. Considered by American Academy of Pediatrics (AAP) to be in category of drugs whose effect on nursing infants is unknown but may be of concern.	11, 17–20
Monoamine oxidase inhibitors (MAOIs)	May inhibit lactation and may interact adversely with tyramine-containing foods; places infant at risk for hypertensive crisis; contraindicated in breast-feeding.	17
Selective serotonin reuptake inhibitors (SSRIs)	Conflicting data. Although some case reports noted no adverse effects, a single case report exists of fluoxetine and norfluoxetine accumulation in an infant's serum and associated colic. U.S. Food and Drug Administration (FDA) has revised its labeling to recommend against use of fluoxetine in nursing women. Single study suggested that sertraline exposure through breast milk caused no adverse effects; sertraline levels in infant were nondetectable.	17, 21–24
bupropion	Bupropion appears to accumulate in breast milk; should be avoided in breast-feeding women.	25
benzodiazepines	Benzodiazepines may accumulate in neonates because of their immature liver enzymes. Diazepam accumulates in breast milk and	17, 26–28

Drug	Description	References
	is not recommended in breast-feeding women. Regular use of other benzodiazepines is best avoided, but occasional doses are unlikely to be harmful. Considered by AAP to be in category of drugs whose effect on nursing infants is unknown but may be of concern.	
Antipsychotics	Except for drowsiness (may occur with chlorpromazine) and galactorrhea (may occur with some phenothiazines), no significant neonatal side effects. Chlorpromazine, haloperidol, mesoridazine are considered by AAP to be in category of drugs whose effect on nursing infants is unknown but may be of concern. One case report exists of clozapine accumulation in breast milk.	17, 26, 28, 29
lithium	Concentration in milk may reach up to 77% of maternal plasma. Because neonatal kidney is immature, risk for lithium accumulation is high. Neonatal cyanosis, T wave abnormalities, hypotonia have been noted in infants breast-fed by mothers taking lithium. AAP considers drug contraindicated during breast-feeding.	17, 26, 28, 30
carbamazepine	Rapidly metabolized, does not appear to accumulate, and therefore may be alternative to lithium use in lactating women. AAP considers drug compatible with breast-feeding.	26, 27
valproic acid	No reported ill effects in breast-fed infants. AAP considers drug compatible with breast-feeding. Because of possibility of hepatotoxicity in infants after drug exposure, however, drug should be used with caution in breast-feeding women.	26, 27

■ REFERENCES

1. Kendell RE, Chalmers JC, Platz C: Epidemiology of puerperal psychoses. Br J Psychiatry 150:662–673, 1987

2. O'Hara MW: Post-partum "blues," depression, and psychosis: a review. J Psychosom Obstet Gynaecol 7:205–227, 1987

3. O'Hara MW: Postpartum depression: causes and consequences. New York, Springer-Verlag, 1995

4. Garvey MJ, Tuason VB, Lumry AE, et al: Occurrence of depression in the postpartum state. J Affect Disord 5:97–101, 1983

5. Wisner KL, Wheeler SB: Prevention of recurrent postpartum major depression. Hosp Community Psychiatry 45:1191–1196, 1994

6. Rohde A, Marneros A: Schizoaffective disorders with and without onset in the puerperium. Eur Arch Psychiatry Clin Neurosci 242:27–33, 1992

7. Davidson J, Robertson E: A follow-up study of postpartum illness, 1946–1978. Acta Psychiatr Scand 71:451–457, 1985

8. Dean C, Williams RJ, Brockington IF: Is puerperal psychosis the same as bipolar manic-depressive disorder? a family study. Psychol Med 19:637–647, 1989

9. Sichel DA: Psychiatric issues in the postpartum period. Currents in Affective Illness 11:5–12, 1992

10. Videbech P, Gouliaev G: First admission with puerperal psychosis: 7–14 years of follow-up. Acta Psychiatr Scand 91:167–173, 1995

11. Stewart DE, Klompenhouwer JL, Kendell RE, et al: Prophylactic lithium in puerperal psychosis. Br J Psychiatry 158:393–397, 1991

12. Gordon JH, Borison RL, Diamond BI: Modulation of dopamine receptor sensitivity by estrogen. Biol Psychiatry 15:389–396, 1980

13. Seeman MV, Lang M: The role of estrogens in schizophrenia gender differences. Schizophr Bull 16:185–194, 1990

14. Kumar R: Postnatal mental illness: a transcultural perspective. Soc Psychiatry Psychiatr Epidemiol 29:250–264, 1994

15. Kruckman LD: Rituals and support: an anthropological view of postpartum depression, in Postpartum Psychiatric Illness: A Picture Puzzle. Edited by Hamilton JA, Harberger PN. Philadelphia, PA, University of Pennsylvania Press, 1992, pp 137–148

16. Goldman AS: The immune system of human milk: antimicrobial, antiinflammatory and immunomodulating properties. Pediatric Infectious Disease Journal 12:664–671, 1993

17. Buist A, Norman TR, Dennerstein L: Breastfeeding and the use of psychotropic medication: a review. J Affect Disord 19:197–206, 1990

18. Misri S, Sivertz K: Tricyclic drugs in pregnancy and lactation: a preliminary report. Int J Psychiatry Med 21:157–171, 1991

19. Matheson I, Pande H, Alertsen AR: Respiratory depression caused by N-desmethyldoxepin in breast milk (letter). Lancet 2:1124, 1985

20. Wisner KL, Perel JM, Foglia JP: Serum clomipramine and metabolite levels in four nursing mother-infant pairs. J Clin Psychiatry 56:17–20, 1995

21. Burch KJ, Wells BG: Fluoxetine/norfluoxetine concentrations in human milk. Pediatrics 89:676–677, 1992

22. Lester BM, Cucca J, Andreozzi BA, et al: Possible association between fluoxetine hydrochloride and colic in an infant. J Am Acad Child Adolesc Psychiatry 32:1253–1255, 1993

23. Nightingale SL: Fluoxetine labeling revised to identify phenytoin interaction and to recommend against use in nursing mothers. JAMA 271:1067, 1994

24. Altshuler LL, Burt VK, McMullen M, et al: Breastfeeding and sertraline: a 24-hour analysis. J Clin Psychiatry 56:243–245, 1995

25. Briggs GC, Samson JH, Ambrose PJ: Excretion of bupropion in breast milk. Ann Pharmacother 27:431–433, 1993

26. American Academy of Pediatrics, Committee on Drugs: Transfer of drugs and other chemicals into human milk. Pediatrics 93:137–150, 1994

27. Beeley L: Drugs and breast-feeding. Clin Obstet Gynecol 13:247–251, 1986

28. Kacew S: Adverse effects of drugs and chemicals in breast milk on the nursing infant. J Clin Pharmacol 33:213–221, 1993

29. Barnas C, Bergant A, Hummer M, et al: Clozapine concentrations in maternal and fetal plasma, amniotic fluid, and breast milk (letter). Am J Psychiatry 151:945, 1994

30. Tunnessen WW, Hertz CG: Toxic effects of lithium in newborn infants: a commentary. J Pediatr 81:804–807, 1972

31. American Academy of Pediatrics, Committee on Drugs: Transfer of drugs and other chemicals into human milk. Pediatrics 93:137–150, 1991

ELECTIVE ABORTION

Elective abortion is the deliberate termination of pregnancy. The landmark U.S. Supreme Court decision *Roe v. Wade* (1973) allowed women to terminate pregnancy in the first trimester, after which period individual state laws prevail. Before and since that time, controversy has raged across the United States regarding a woman's right to choose abortion. In this chapter we discuss the medical and psychological issues associated with elective abortion.

■ EPIDEMIOLOGY

6

Each year, about 1.5 million abortions (344 abortions per 1,000 live births) are performed in the United States. In the United States, most women who elect to have an abortion are single and under 25 and have not had previous live births. In developing nations, most women who have elective abortions are married and have several children.

Over the past 20 years, the percentage of pregnancies ending in abortion has dropped steadily, possibly because of attitudinal changes toward elective abortion, increased use of contraception, reduced access to abortion services, and a decline in unplanned pregnancies. In the years since *Roe v. Wade,* the proportion of teenagers obtaining abortions has decreased, but it has increased for women over 40; 51% of pregnancies in the over-40 population are electively terminated.

A total of 88.4% of elective abortions are performed within the first trimester of pregnancy, and 99% are performed before the 21st week (1). A 1987 survey of abortion patients across the United States found that half were practicing contraception during the month in which they conceived (2). The patients who did not use contraception were more likely to be young, poor, black or Hispanic, and less educated than users of contraception.

■ ABORTION TECHNIQUES AND MORTALITY AND MORBIDITY

The abortion method for 90% of all abortions is dilatation of the cervix and evacuation of the uterine contents by means of vacuum aspiration or curettage. First-trimester abortions and most second-trimester abortions are accomplished by this means.

The mortality rate from elective abortion is approximately 0.4 per 100,000 procedures. Risk factors include older maternal age, non-Caucasian race, older gestational age, and techniques of abortion other than curettage. Notably, the rate of mortality from childbirth is 25 times greater than that from elective abortion. Although the years since 1940 have been characterized by a decline in deaths due to both childbirth and abortion, the abortion mortality ratio for women (abortions per 1,000 live births) has declined more rapidly than has maternal mortality. The steepest drop in women's mortality due to abortion has occurred since 1967–1970, the years corresponding to the liberalization of state abortion laws.

Induced abortion is not associated with an increased risk of subsequent infertility. Additionally, prior elective abortion has no effect on the rate of subsequent pregnancy-related morbidity, including spontaneous abortion, premature delivery, and low-birth-weight infants (3).

■ REASONS FOR ELECTIVE ABORTION

Women elect to have an abortion for a number of reasons. They include an inability to support a child financially, lack of willingness or ability to assume the responsibility for a child, lack of social supports, impregnation by incest or rape, reluctance to be a single parent, conflicts with a partner, and diagnosis of a fetal congenital anomaly.

■ PRENATAL DIAGNOSIS AND ELECTIVE ABORTION

Prenatal diagnostic tests are used for a variety of reasons, including dating of the pregnancy, assessment of fetal anomalies, location of the placenta, and determination of amniotic fluid volume. When prenatal tests reveal serious congenital anomalies, consideration is usually given to termination of the pregnancy. If a decision is made to continue with the pregnancy, knowledge prior to the delivery allows time to adjust to a difficult outcome. Indications and timing for prenatal diagnostic tests are described in Table 6–1.

■ PSYCHOLOGICAL EFFECTS OF ELECTIVE ABORTION

An undesired pregnancy is a major crisis in a woman's life that is often resolved by termination of the pregnancy. Structured tests to evaluate mood and well-being in women have shown improved scores immediately following abortion and for years thereafter (4).

Although most women experience few or no adverse psychological sequelae after an elective abortion, some women do experience postabortion psychological distress. Factors increasing the likelihood of negative emotional experiences include medical or genetic indications for the abortion, a psy-

TABLE 6-1. Prenatal diagnostic tests: indications, timing, and risk of fetal loss

Test	Indications	Timing	Fetal loss rate (%)
Maternal serum analyte screening: assays for maternal serum α-fetoprotein (MSAFP), human chorionic gonadotropin (HCG), unconjugated estriol (uE$_3$)	All patients: to screen for incorrect dating, multiple gestation, neural tube defects, certain fetal chromosomal abnormalities (e.g., trisomy 21, trisomy 18), other fetal anomalies, fetal death	15–20 weeks of gestation	0
Fetal ultrasound	Level I (basic) ultrasound: uncertain gestational age, location and grade of placenta, number of fetuses, cardiac activity, amniotic fluid volume, vaginal bleeding, detection of gross fetal abnormalities	Varies: early in first trimester or any other time	0
	Level II (targeted) ultrasound: previous fetus or infant with congenital anomaly, family history of congenital anomaly, in utero exposure to any potential teratogen (e.g., valproic acid, carbamazepine, lithium)	18–20 weeks of gestation	0

Amniocentesis	Maternal age at least 35 years, abnormal maternal serum analyte screening, history of chromosomal anomaly in fetus or infant, chromosomal abnormality in parent, family history of detectable Mendelian disorder	12–15 weeks of gestation	1–2
		15–20 weeks of gestation	0.5–1.0
Chorionic villus sampling	Maternal age at least 35 years, history of chromosomal anomaly in previous fetus or infant, chromosomal abnormality in parent, family history of detectable Mendelian disorder, history of 3 or more spontaneous abortions	9–13 weeks of gestation	0.5–1.5

chiatric history, an abortion performed at mid-trimester (especially if induction of labor and delivery was required for termination of the pregnancy), ambivalence about the decision to abort, and a feeling that the decision was not freely made (4).

■ ABORTION COUNSELING

Abortion counseling is an important component of the abortion procedure. Having an abortion is a momentous event for most women, and counseling is an opportunity to assess available options, screen for psychological difficulties or serious psychopathology, provide information regarding the abortion procedure, and review ways to prevent future unplanned pregnancies. Counseling also gives women an opportunity to express and assimilate feelings connected with the relationship in which pregnancy occurred and issues connected with abortion as a possible outcome. For women who choose abortion, counseling minimizes preoperative anxiety and hastens postoperative recovery.

Many women who consider abortion have questions about the procedure and mixed feelings about their choice. It is important that the setting for abortion be both medically safe and psychologically supportive. It is both common and understandable for women to have concerns about the safety of abortion, the extent of pain and discomfort present during or after the procedure, and possible sequelae. In this regard, abortion counseling—besides offering psychological support— provides information about the procedure itself and about possible complications. For this reason, the abortion counselor should understand reproductive physiology and be knowledgeable about abortion procedures.

For the most part, first-trimester patients tend to experience less stress than do second-trimester patients. This second group are more likely to be young, poor, and unfamiliar with gynecological procedures (5). All patients should be given the opportunity to discuss their reasons for considering an abortion. For patients who are ambivalent or who present for abortion to satisfy parents or a partner, but who have not truly explored what they want for themselves, it is essential to provide an open opportunity for discussion of the alternatives available to pregnant women.

Although most women who have abortions do not experience negative psychological sequelae, some experience a heightened awareness of interpersonal or other difficulties in their lives. Many women who decide to proceed with abortion do not want and do not require further counseling after the abortion. Nevertheless, it is useful at least to offer options for ongoing counseling should the patient request further assistance.

The Process of Abortion Counseling

The patient who presents for abortion counseling should be encouraged to examine her feelings concerning the pregnancy, the prospect of abortion, the relationship in which the pregnancy occurred, and possible feelings after the abortion has been completed. The basic anatomy and physiology of reproduction should be reviewed, and the abortion procedure itself should be discussed. The patient should be aware of how to obtain follow-up assistance, both medical and psychological, should these be needed. Options for subsequent birth control should be carefully discussed and the risks and benefits of each alternative reviewed.

Women whose pregnancy results from rape are likely to experience psychological difficulties because they are pregnant and also because they have been raped. Although abortion counseling is an appropriate and necessary part of the mental health process, these patients often require additional mental health care, for they are likely to experience psychological sequelae as a result of their traumatic experience. As with all women who present for abortion, feelings should be explored. Information about the procedure and its risks and possible complications should be reviewed. Provision should be made for follow-up rape crisis counseling.

Another difficult situation presenting in the setting of abortion counseling is that of the woman who requests an abortion because of a severe fetal deformity or impending fetal death. Such women should be given ample opportunity to express their feelings. Following the decision to abort an abnormal fetus, women may experience mourning for the loss of a wished-for baby, and they often benefit from bereavement counseling. In some cases, guilt for having produced a deformed fetus may require sensitive exploration and resolution (6). Decision making about subsequent pregnancies may be fraught with ambivalence, fear, and anxiety, and women may need close follow-up with mental health professionals over the course of future pregnancies. The clinician must be patient and empathic. Communication between the mental health counselor and the obstetrician is essential so that reassurance and support are given by clinicians who fully understand the obstetrical complications encountered by the patient. Also included in the therapy should be the woman's partner, who may also be grieving, but who may come to be relied on as a source of support for the pregnant partner rather than as a person in need of psychological support. Providing abortion counseling requires a team effort. Ideally, the team includes the patient, her partner, the gynecologist, and a skilled and sensitive mental health counselor with knowledge of reproductive physiology and abortion procedure.

The pregnant woman with a chronic mental illness presents special issues for the abortion counselor. Assessment of the psychotic pregnant woman should be performed by an experienced psychiatrist. Evaluation should address ongoing delusions, paranoia, and hallucinations. The ability of the patient to understand her pregnant condition and to appreciate fully all feasible options should be assessed. Management of the pregnant psychotic patient should first be directed toward stabilization of her psychiatric condition. For patients whose condition presents a danger to either themselves or their unborn babies, it is invariably necessary to institute involuntary hospitalization. Collateral support from the partner and family members should be elicited. Once the patient is stabilized, management issues related to continuation or termination of the pregnancy can be addressed.

■ REFERENCES

1. Frye AA, Atrash HK, Lawson HW, et al: Induced abortion in the United States: a 1994 update. J Am Med Wom Assoc 49:131–136, 1994
2. Henshaw SK, Silverman J: The characteristics and prior contraceptive use of U.S. abortion patients. Fam Plann Perspect 20:158–168, 1988
3. Frank PI, Kay CR, Scott LM, et al: Pregnancy following induced abortion: maternal morbidity, congenital abnormalities and neonatal death. Br J Obstet Gynaecol 94:836–842, 1987
4. Dagg PKB: The psychological sequelae of therapeutic abortion—denied and completed. Am J Psychiatry 148:578–585, 1991
5. Hern WM: Abortion counseling, in Abortion Practice. Philadelphia, PA, JB Lippincott, 1990, p 77
6. Zolese G, Blacker CVR: The psychological complications of therapeutic abortion. Br J Psychiatry 160:742–749, 1992

INFERTILITY: PSYCHOLOGICAL IMPLICATIONS OF DIAGNOSIS AND TREATMENT

■ EPIDEMIOLOGY

Infertility is defined as the inability of a couple to achieve pregnancy after at least 1 year of unprotected intercourse. In the United States, 2.4 million couples, or 10%–15% of all couples in the country, experience infertility (1). Since the 1970s, the number of office visits to physicians for infertility consultation has more than doubled. More than $1.3 billion is spent on the diagnosis and treatment of infertility due solely to pelvic inflammatory disease (2). That cost does not include the large numbers of health care dollars spent on assisted reproductive technologies (i.e., techniques involving direct retrieval of oocytes from the ovary) (Table 7–1).

■ ETIOLOGY

Infertility may be secondary to a male factor, a female factor, or a combination of factors contributed by both members of a couple (Table 7–2). Historically, women were thought to bear the sole responsibility for infertility; today it is believed that

7

TABLE 7–1.   **Epidemiology of infertility (1988)**

8.4% of women ages 15–44 (4.9 million women) have impaired
   fertility (55% have at least one child, 45% have never had
   children).

25% of women have an episode of infertility at some point during
   their reproductive life.

43% of infertile couples seek medical assistance.

4.6% of married women consult a physician for impaired fertility.

24% of infertile women receive treatment (tubal surgery,
   insemination, ovulation induction, or in vitro fertilization).

Approximately 50% of infertile couples eventually conceive.

Source.   Data adapted from Jones and Toner 1993 (3).

TABLE 7–2.   **Etiological factors in infertility**

Contributing factor	% of cases
Male factor	40–60
Ovulatory dysfunction	30
Uterine or tubal disease	20
Cervical problems, immunological factors, infectious diseases	5
Unexplained	20

Source.   Reprinted from McCartney CF, Downey J: "New Reproductive
Technologies," in *Medical Psychiatric Practice.* Edited by Stoudemire A, Fogel
PS. Washington, DC, American Psychiatric Press, 1993, p. 302. Used with
permission.

male factors contribute to 40%–60% of infertility and that
more than one cause contributes to infertility in 10%–30% of
couples (3, 4). Up to 10% of infertility may be partially or
completely explained by premature ejaculation and impotence
(5). Psychological factors contributing to infertility include
anorexia nervosa and unconsummated sexual relationships.
Although there are intricate feedback loops that may indirectly
control the neuroendocrine pathways impinging on fertility,
the current consensus does not suggest that psychiatric syn-

dromes play a significant role in infertility. Although some studies suggest differences in psychological profile between infertile and fertile persons, it is likely that infertility is the cause rather than the result of these differences (6).

■ RELATED PSYCHOLOGICAL FACTORS

For most couples, infertility is a significant life crisis. Infertile couples pass through a series of phases, including disbelief, denial, frustration, anger, grief, and eventually acceptance. For couples who choose to investigate possible causes and then to proceed to treatment, huge monetary costs add to the stress they experience.

Although infertility clearly affects the marital relationship, for some couples the relationship is actually strengthened, possibly because the couple share in the experience of decision making and in participation in treating the problem.

Psychological Factors for the Woman

Infertile women tend to feel frustrated and less feminine and to suffer from decreased self-esteem (7). A study of women in the initial stages of infertility treatment and evaluation revealed that although they were clearly emotionally distressed by their inability to have children, their distress did not result in psychological impairment (8). Nevertheless, women with infertility report high levels of psychological distress, dysphoria, a decline in their sexual functioning, and a feeling of lowered self-worth. In many cases, infertile women feel that the issue of their infertility has become so all-important to them that they are less interested in other aspects of their lives (8).

When a couple is faced with infertility, women tend to be more emotionally affected than their male partners (9). This tendency appears to be true at the point of initial diagnosis and after years of treatment.

Psychological Factors for the Man

Although women tend to be more psychologically affected than their partners when faced with the inability to conceive, some men nevertheless show signs of considerable anxiety, either because infertility results in part or fully from a male factor or because treatment requires performance by the man in a scheduled manner. Particularly for men with anxious personalities, the demands of sexual performance during the fertile portion of the menstrual cycle make it difficult or impossible to sustain an erection. It is sometimes difficult or even impossible for men to produce a semen sample for the postcoital examination or for intrauterine insemination. For men, as for women, self-esteem is often closely connected to the ability to perform sexually.

Psychological Factors Shared by the Couple

Infertile couples often feel socially isolated, particularly when their peers are occupied with child-rearing and organize their social activities around their children. In an effort to avoid painful questioning about their childlessness or future plans, such couples may avoid family gatherings. The financial burden of both evaluation and treatment for infertility is an additional significant source of stress and may mean alterations in financial decisions, such as the purchase of a home or a car or taking vacations. Not uncommonly, couples will turn to credit cards to finance expensive technological approaches, even when the likelihood of their success is poor. Infertile women undergoing assisted reproductive technological treatment may postpone or refuse career advancement opportunities because of the physical and logistic demands entailed by the treatment.

■ EVALUATION

The workup for infertility is both comprehensive and extensive and often involves evaluation of both partners (Table 7–3). The infertility workup includes baseline evaluations for general health, screening for sexually transmitted diseases and normal endocrine functioning, assessment of ovulation, assessment of the quantity and quality of sperm, visualization of the woman's anatomy, and determination of the patency of ductile systems in the woman and/or the man. Tests are often repeated at intervals over a single menstrual cycle and at subsequent menstrual cycles. The assessment invariably requires substantial reorganization of the day-to-day lives of both partners, because office visits are dictated by responses to treatment, dates of ovulation, and physicians' schedules.

One of the first studies in an infertility assessment is daily basal body temperature recording for at least 1 or 2 months. Each morning before rising, the woman records her body temperature. A temperature rise occurs in response to ovulation and the increase in the level of progesterone. The days when intercourse have occurred are also recorded. Another early study, the postcoital test, involves a sampling of cervical mucus collected from a woman within 8 hours after intercourse. The couple is instructed not to have intercourse for 1–2 days before the sampling. The sample is then assayed for its suitability as an

---

TABLE 7–3. **Diagnostic studies to evaluate infertility**

Comprehensive medical, surgical, reproductive history of both partners

Physical examination of both partners

Endocrine evaluations: both partners

Basal body temperature charting; recording of dates of intercourse

Semen analysis

Postcoital test

Endometrial biopsy

Hysterosalpingogram

Laparoscopy

Tests of patency of male ductile system

---

environment for sperm and for the quantity and quality of motile sperm. Although these diagnostic tests appear rather simple, they involve sharing the details of sexual acts with medical personnel, who often "medicalize" the natural and personal components of an intimate physical relationship. Men frequently have performance anxiety, and both men and women may feel frustrated, irritable, anxious, and angry.

Early in the evaluation for infertility, the man collects semen by masturbation. Although technically simple, the process is difficult for many men, who are sometimes unable to perform on command in the setting of a medical office.

The semen is analyzed microscopically to confirm adequate volume, viscosity, pH, sperm count, motility, and morphology and to rule out infectious agents such as *Ureaplasma* and *Mycoplasma.*

For the woman whose cervical mucus appears to be normal and who is ovulating regularly but is nevertheless unable to conceive, a hysterosalpingogram is often performed. This examination, which visualizes any mechanical blockage to sperm, involves the injection of radiopaque dye into the female reproductive tract. A side effect may involve transient pelvic cramping. Laparoscopy, involving direct visualization of the female reproductive organs by insertion of a laparoscope through the navel (with the patient under general anesthesia), may also be performed to rule out anatomic abnormalities. General anesthesia will become less common in the future; it will be replaced by conscious sedation. An endometrial biopsy, generally performed late in the menstrual cycle, confirms ovulation and the production of adequate hormones after ovulation.

■ TREATMENT

Whenever possible, infertility treatment is aimed at reversing pathology isolated by assessment studies (see Table 7–4). When hysterosalpingography or laparoscopy reveals mechanical blockage or anatomical abnormalities (40%–50% of cases of female infertility), treatment is directed at removing the defect. In some cases, adhesions from endometriosis may be removed through the laparoscope. Gonadotropin-releasing hormone (GnRH) agonists such as leuprolide acetate (Lupron), goserelin (Zoladex), and nafarelin acetate (Synarel) are the treatments of choice for endometriosis. Any of these treatments may cause depression or emotional lability.

In cases of ovulatory dysfunction, induction of ovulation is attempted initially with orally administered clomiphene citrate, a nonsteroidal antiestrogen. Psychiatric side effects of clomiphene include depression, nervousness, and insomnia. If, after several attempts, ovulation has not been successfully induced by clomiphene citrate, human menopausal gonadotropins are often administered by daily injections. (Medications used are either menotropins [Pergonal], a combination of follicle-stimulating hormone and luteinizing hormone [FSH/LH], or urofollitropin [Metrodin] [FSH].) Injections may be performed

TABLE 7–4. **Conventional treatments for infertility**

Cause of infertility	Treatment
Ovulatory failure	Clomiphene citrate, pulsatile GnRH (pump) administration, gonadotropin
Tubal damage	Tubal operations
Semen factor	None, donor or intrauterine insemination
Endometriosis	Ablation
Cervical factor	Intrauterine insemination
Luteal-phase deficiency	Correction of cause, progesterone, or clomiphene citrate
Unexplained	Clomiphene citrate, gonadotropin, intrauterine insemination

Note. GnRH = gonadotropin-releasing hormone.
Source. Jones HW, Toner JP: "The infertile couple." *N Engl J Med* 329:1710–1715, 1993. Copyright 1993, Massachusetts Medical Society. Reprinted by permission of *The New England Journal of Medicine.*

by the woman herself or her partner, or she may want to make daily visits to her physician for administration of the drug. Side effects may include fatigue, nausea, headache, diarrhea, and weight gain. The likelihood of multiple gestation (usually twins) is increased to 5% with clomiphene citrate and 20% with human menopausal gonadotropins. Throughout the procedure, serial ultrasounds confirm normal ovulation and monitor follicular development. In some cases, pulsatile administration of GnRH may be used to induce ovulation.

When infertility persists after conventional therapy, or when fallopian tubes are irreversibly obstructed or damaged, infertile couples are treated with assisted reproductive technology (see Table 7–5). This term includes techniques that involve retrieving oocytes directly from the ovary. Embryos or gametes are then transferred directly into the woman. Ovulation is induced by injections of gonadotropin, and oocytes are retrieved. In gamete intrafallopian transfer (GIFT), oocytes and sperm are immediately placed in the fallopian tubes. In zygote intrafallopian transfer (ZIFT), fertilized embryos are placed in the tubes 1-2 days after retrieval. For in vitro fertilization (IVF), fertilized embryos are placed directly into the uterine cavity. Serial ultrasounds are administered and estradiol levels are assayed to monitor ovulation and posttransfer development and to rule out ovarian hyperstimulation. These procedures are exceedingly expensive—thousands of dollars per attempt—and most couples are advised to make three to four attempts. Because multiple gametes or zygotes are often transferred at

TABLE 7–5. **Assisted reproduction**	
Modality	**% success rate (1989)**
In vitro fertilization (IVF)	14
Gamete intrafallopian transfer (GIFT)	23
Zygote intrafallopian transfer (ZIFT)	15

Source. Data from McCartney and Downey 1993 (4), p. 309.

one time, assisted reproductive technology increases the probability of multiple gestation to about 25%. There is also a 6% chance of severe ovarian hyperstimulation syndrome, a potentially life-threatening complication. Intraooplasmic sperm injection followed by artificial insemination is now used for severe male factor infertility.

In the case of multiple gestation, there is an increased risk of medical complications, pregnancy loss, and increased expense, as well as the difficulties of raising more than one child.

When infertility is due to a male factor that is not treatable, artificial insemination by a donor (AID), also called therapeutic donor insemination (TDI), is a technically simple and highly successful modality. Receiving a donated egg is a useful strategy for the woman who is unable to ovulate even with medical assistance. This process is more complex than AID, for it involves treatment of the donor and the infertile woman with medications to synchronize their cycles. By means of IVF or GIFT, donor eggs are fertilized with sperm and the infertile woman is inseminated and carries the pregnancy. A final, more controversial treatment involves the use of a surrogate mother to carry the fertilized egg of a woman who is able to ovulate but not to carry a pregnancy successfully.

■ PSYCHOLOGICAL REACTIONS TO INFERTILITY TREATMENT

Infertility treatment—with its stress of constant monitoring of reproduction-related bodily functions, need to regulate intimate sexual acts, and expenditure of large sums of money with no guarantee of success—provides a setting for the possible emergence of dysphoria and anxiety (Table 7–6). Many of the agents used in infertility treatment protocols affect the hypothalamic-pituitary-ovarian and have the potential of fairly powerful physical and psychological side effects.

TABLE 7–6.	**Adverse impact of infertility and infertility procedures**

Depression, anxiety, hostility (women > men)

Negative impact on sexual functioning: impotence, anorgasmia, decreased libido

Social isolation

Financial difficulties

Unrealistic expectations of outcome of pregnancy

Multiple births

For some women, in addition to the physiological side effects on mood caused by these agents, mood swings occur as a reaction to the stress of pursuing conception over the course of many months. Thus, hope and anxiety increase in the days before ovulation and as the projected date of menses nears. With the arrival of the menses, signaling that gestation has not occurred, depressive symptoms surface.

Partners often find that in synchronizing their sexual acts with the needs of the fertility treatment, the spontaneity of their sexual relationship is lost. This loss may result in an inability to perform on the part of either the husband, who may be unable to maintain an erection or to ejaculate, or the wife—who may suffer from vaginismus or dyspareunia. Where multiple gestation occurs, pregnancy is often difficult and increases the risk of premature births of babies with multiple medical problems. Often, when a couple has been infertile for a number of years and has been single-mindedly devoted to achieving pregnancy through assisted reproductive technology, little thought is given to the realities of child-rearing. Paradoxically, such parents may be faced with a letdown when they achieve their goal of becoming parents.

Women who have postponed childbearing to accomplish career aspirations are often used to maintaining control over their lives and achieving carefully planned goals. When these women discover that they are unsuccessful at achieving pregnancy, they feel frustrated and angry because they are now faced with a situation over which they have no control. Guilt because of conscious past decisions to postpone conception or to undergo prior therapeutic abortions is not uncommon.

■ TREATMENT OF PSYCHOLOGICAL DIFFICULTIES RELATED TO INFERTILITY

Frequently, infertility specialists refer an infertile woman for psychiatric assessment before beginning or continuing her treatment for infertility. For patients who have had continuous treatment without success, a treatment holiday may be helpful to allow a couple to return to a more natural routine without the dictates of medical intervention. This holiday period also allows time to reevaluate alternative options. Even if one member of a couple is more disabled psychiatrically than the other, it is often very helpful to see both members of the couple for at least several sessions. RESOLVE, the national self-help organization for infertile couples, sponsors support groups throughout the United States that are often very helpful in destigmatizing the issue of infertility and enabling couples to feel both strengthened and less isolated.

Although infertile women are no more likely to develop a major depressive or anxiety disorder than are the general population of women, in some cases the stress of diagnosis and treatment may cause or exacerbate psychiatric disorders. For mild to moderate psychiatric symptoms, psychotherapy may be all that is necessary. For major mood or anxiety disorders, treatment should involve psychotherapy and/or psychotropic medication. The use of medications to induce ovulation or sustain gestation may complicate treatment, for many of these agents may exacerbate psychiatric difficulties or reduce the effectiveness of psychotropic medications. Collaborative discussions should include the psychiatrist, the couple, and the treating infertility specialist. The psychiatrist may provide a supportive environment in which to realistically review the probability of achieving success with further infertility treatments. Empathic psychotherapy to explore alternative options, including postponement of infertility treatments, adoption, and discussion of ways other than parenting to derive gratification for caregiving aspirations, may also be explored. Should the couple decide to move ahead with further infertility treatments, the psychiatrist may then provide ongoing support and treatment (Table 7–7).

■ WHEN THE INFERTILE COUPLE SUCCEEDS IN ACHIEVING PREGNANCY

For the couple whose energy has been focused for years on the achievement of a successful impregnation, the realization of a long-awaited biological child is invariably met with great joy and relief. It is not unusual, however, for the previously infertile couple to encounter significant difficulties with their new roles as parents. In trying to achieve pregnancy, the husband and wife may have neglected to anticipate their roles as parents

---

TABLE 7–7. **Roles for psychiatry in the treatment of infertility**

Performing a psychiatric evaluation

Helping patients to clarify issues, gain insight into motivations, make choice that best serves their interests

Helping patients with decision-making

Helping partners reach consensus

Helping patients cope with stresses of infertility treatments

Providing treatment holidays

Referring for individual supportive therapy

Referring to support groups (see Appendix)

Providing psychopharmacological treatment

Source. Adapted from McCartney and Downey 1993 (4).

of a child whose presence means renegotiating their relationship as husband and wife. Additionally, as a woman's body grows over the 9 months of pregnancy, the couple's triumph over the long years during which they felt inadequate in comparison to their peers may be so great that they have difficulty in letting go of the increasingly visible pregnant state.

For many infertile couples who have been in psychotherapy, it is therefore helpful to continue in therapy over the course of pregnancy and through at least the first 6 months of parenthood. In a supportive psychotherapeutic setting, both husband and wife will have the opportunity to explore their relationship apart from issues related to fertility, sexual performance on command, or connections with medical personnel. Reevaluating the emotional bonds that connected them long before they were aware of fertility difficulties may be important for the couple as they await and anticipate the birth of their child.

■ REFERENCES

1. LaPane KL, Zierler S, Lasater TM, et al: Is a history of depressive symptoms associated with an increased risk of infertility in women? Psychosom Med 57:509–513, 1995
2. Cates W, Rolfs RT, Aral SO: Sexually transmitted diseases, pelvic inflammatory disease, and infertility: an epidemiology update. Epidemiology Review 12:199–220, 1990
3. Jones HW, Toner JP: The infertile couple. N Engl J Med 23:1710–1715, 1993
4. McCartney CF, Downey J: New reproductive technologies, in Medical Psychiatric Practice. Edited by Stoudemire A, Fogel PS. Washington, DC, American Psychiatric Press, 1993, p 302
5. Seibel MM, Taymor ML: Emotional aspects of infertility. Fertil Steril 37:137–145, 1982
6. Stotland NL, Smith TE: Psychiatric consultation to obstetrics and gynecology: systems and syndromes, in American Psychiatric Press Review of Psychiatry, Vol 9. Edited by Tasman A, Goldfinger SM,

Kaufmann CA. Washington, DC, American Psychiatric Press, 1990, pp 537–563

7. Facchinetti F, Demyttenaere K, Fioroni L, et al: Psychosomatic disorders related to gynecology. Psychother Psychosom 58:137–154, 1992

8. Downey J, McKinney M: The psychiatric status of women presenting for infertility evaluation. Am J Orthopsychiatry 62:196–205, 1992

9. Downey J: Infertility and the new reproductive technologies, in Psychological Aspects of Women's Health Care: The Interface Between Psychiatry and Obstetrics and Gynecology. Edited by Stewart DE, Stotland NL. Washington, DC, American Psychiatric Press, 1993, pp 193–206

PERIMENOPAUSE AND MENOPAUSE

■ DEFINITIONS AND HISTORY

Menopause is the point at which a woman has permanently ceased menstruating. *Perimenopause,* typically occurring 5–7 years before menopause, is the interval between regular ovulatory menstrual cycles and complete cessation of ovarian function. The *climacteric* is a general term used to describe the years of declining ovarian function.

Until recently, menopause was thought to be a time of moodiness, irritability, and somatization. In 1890, Kraepelin coined the term *involutional melancholia* for a syndrome of agitated depression, hypochondriasis, and nihilistic delusions in menopausal women. This syndrome was included as a diagnostic category in DSM-I (1) and DSM-II (2). Because extensive epidemiological data collected in the 1970s found no evidence for the diagnosis, it was dropped from DSM-III (3).

Natural menopause occurs between the ages of 44 and 55 (average 51.4 years). Because women today live to an average age of 81 years, the menopausal years can make up more than one-third of a woman's life. Most women experience physiological changes during the perimenopausal and menopausal years, and some may additionally experience mood alterations.

8

■ HORMONAL CHANGES

During perimenopause, when ovarian function and fertility are declining, there may be few signs of the decline. The interval between menstrual periods may shorten or lengthen, and menstrual bleeding may become lighter or heavier. Occasionally a period is skipped, and this generally corresponds to a month when ovulation has not occurred. As menopause is approached, menstrual periods become progressively lighter and more infrequent, then cease completely.

In response to decreased estrogen production by the ovary, the pituitary hormones luteinizing hormone (LH) and follicle-stimulating hormone (FSH) rise. The ovarian hormone inhibin, which negatively feeds back to decrease FSH release, also decreases, contributing to the rise in FSH. An elevated serum FSH level, taken on day 2 or 3 after the onset of menses, suggests a woman is perimenopausal. Elevated FSH levels obtained later in the cycle can be misleading, because this hormone may rise into the menopausal range in premenopausal women, particularly at midcycle (Figure 2–2). At and after menopause, levels of estradiol, the biologically active form of estrogen, remain under 25 pg/mL, and levels of FSH remain over 40 mIU/mL.

■ PHYSICAL CHANGES

The physical signs and symptoms of perimenopause and menopause result from declining estrogen production. Vasomotor symptoms, including hot flashes and cold sweats, occur in 80% of perimenopausal women. These symptoms may persist for several years beyond the last menstrual period. Hot flashes are sensations of extreme heat that develop unexpectedly in the face, upper body, or entire body and last for 1–5 minutes. They are followed by sweating and a feeling of cold as perspiration evaporates. Breathlessness, dizziness, and an increased heart rate may occur. Because these symptoms are not unlike those of panic attacks, the differential diagnosis of new-onset panic disorder in the middle-aged woman should include perimenopausal vasomotor symptoms. When vasomotor symptoms occur at night, a woman may experience insomnia and the subsequent effects of sleep deprivation, including decreased concentration, fatigue, and irritability. Hot flashes often occur when women are still menstruating.

The decline in ovarian estrogen production is associated with a number of physical changes. They include atrophy of the urogenital tract lining, sometimes resulting in atrophic inflammation of the vagina and urinary tract. Infection and dyspareunia may result, with subsequent urinary frequency, urgency, and occasional stress incontinence. Osteoporosis and cardiovascular disease are long-term consequences of low estrogen levels.

■ MOOD CHANGES

In general, longitudinal studies have not found that natural menopause increases the risk for depression in most women (4, 5). However, some women may experience depressive symptomatology at menopause. In particular, women who suffer severe vasomotor symptoms (hot flashes, night sweats) appear to be at risk for depressive symptomatology. As their physical symptoms resolve, mood symptoms return to baseline. Also at risk for psychological complaints at menopause are women with histories of reproduction-related mood syndromes, including oral-contraceptive–related mood complaints, premenstrual dysphoria, and postpartum depression (6). Health problems and social stressors also increase the risk of depressive symptoms in perimenopausal women. Being divorced, widowed, or separated, having a lower level of education, and experiencing stress from caretaking responsibilities appear to be related to depression during menopause (7, 8). Interestingly, neither death of parents nor children leaving the home seems to be a risk factor for the development of depression at this time (4). Depression in women before perimenopause increases the likelihood of depression during the perimenopausal years (Table 8–1).

■ MENOPAUSE AND SEXUALITY

Most women who have been sexually active before menopause remain so during the perimenopausal years. Nevertheless, physiological changes resulting from estrogen decline may produce decreased sexual responsiveness and libido. Atrophic urogenital tract changes may result in vaginal dryness, infection, and subsequent dyspareunia. Estrogen replacement, in the form of oral supplementation, vaginal cream, or skin patches, is often effective treatment for urogenital atrophic changes. For women whose main symptom is diminished libido, small amounts of testosterone supplementation may be helpful (9, 10).

Sexual dysfunction cannot always be attributed to perimenopausal urogenital changes. Other factors that may impair sexual function include chronic health problems, depression, relationship conflicts, or partner sexual dysfunction. The as-

---

TABLE 8–1. **Factors associated with development of depression in the menopausal transition**

History of depression

History of oral-contraceptive–related dysphoria

History of premenstrual dysphoric disorder

History of postpartum depression

Severe vasomotor symptoms

Caretaking responsibilities

Lower level of education

Loss of significant other (widowhood, divorce, separation)

Chronic health problems

---

sessment of sexual functioning should therefore address psychological and social issues in addition to physical symptoms (Table 8–2).

■ HORMONE REPLACEMENT THERAPY

Treatment Regimens

Hormone replacement for women with an intact uterus generally requires the administration of estrogen and progestin. The progestin is prescribed to counteract the risk of endometrial cancer associated with unopposed estrogen. Hormone replacement in women who have had a hysterectomy therefore does not require progestin in addition to estrogen.

For women with an intact uterus, hormone replacement therapy is instituted either cyclically or continuously. Although strategies for hormone replacement may vary among clinicians, estrogen is typically given every day of the month, and progestin is provided either on days 1–12 of each month (cyclic regimen) or on every day of the month (continuous regimen). The advantage of the cyclic regimen is that women may reliably expect vaginal bleeding in the days following withdrawal of progestin. Bleeding at any other time of the month is unwarranted and requires gynecological assessment and endometrial biopsy to rule out endometrial hyperplasia or malignancy. The

TABLE 8–2.	Possible causes of sexual dysfunction in perimenopausal women

Urogenital changes related to estrogen deficiency

Chronic health problems

Poor physical fitness

Depression

Unsatisfactory premenopausal sexual function

Sexual dysfunction in the partner

continuous regimen has the advantage of freedom from monthly bleeding, but occasional spotting may occur, particularly during the first year of hormone replacement. Endometrial biopsies may thus be required to rule out endometrial hyperplasia or malignancy.

Doses of estrogen and progestin vary with preparations (Table 8–3). Common dosage preparations are conjugated equine estrogen (Premarin) 0.625 mg daily and medroxyprogesterone acetate (Provera) 2.5 mg daily throughout the month or 5–10 mg on days 1–12.

Risks and Benefits

Estrogen effectively treats the vasomotor symptoms of hot flashes and associated sleep disturbance. Urogenital atrophy is also improved with estrogen therapy. When evaluating other effects of estrogen replacement therapy, it is important to understand that coronary heart disease is the leading cause of

TABLE 8–3. **Common doses and preparations of estrogen and progestin**

Formulation	Dose (mg)
Estrogen preparations	
conjugated equine estrogen	0.3, 0.625, 1.25
piperazine estrone sulfate	0.6, 1.2
micronized estradiol	1, 2
estradiol valerate	1, 2
conjugated estrogen vaginal cream	1.25, 2.5
transdermal estradiol patch	0.05, 0.1
progestin preparations	
medroxyprogesterone acetate	2.5, 5, 10
megestrol acetate	20, 40
norethindrone	0.35, 5
norethindrone acetate	5
norgestrel	0.075
micronized progesterone	100

death in postmenopausal women and that osteoporosis is a widespread and disabling disease in older women. Although breast cancer is a serious and life-threatening disease, the median age at which it develops is 69 years. For a 50-year-old woman, the lifetime probability of developing cardiovascular disease is five times greater than that for breast cancer (11) (Table 8–4).

Estrogen replacement reduces the relative risk of disabling osteoporotic hip fracture to 0.75 and of cardiovascular disease to 0.55–0.65 (11). Data are not yet sufficient to determine the effect of progestin supplementation on the benefits of estrogen replacement (12). For many women, particularly those at high risk for coronary heart disease and osteoporosis, hormone replacement therapy is likely to improve both quality and length of life.

For women with an intact uterus, estrogen replacement causes an eightfold increase in the risk of endometrial cancer after 1–2 decades of use (11). This risk is obliterated with the addition of progestin. Although some studies suggest that there is an increase in breast cancer among women who have taken estrogen for more than 5 years, other studies do not support this finding (12). The effect of progestin supplementation on the risk of breast cancer is controversial (13). In women at high

TABLE 8–4. **Probability of breast cancer, osteoporotic hip fracture, and coronary heart disease in 50-year-old women**

Disease	Lifetime probability for a 50-year-old woman (%)	Probability of dying from disease (%)
Breast cancer	10	3
Osteoporotic hip fracture	15	1.5
Coronary heart disease	46	31

Source. Data from Grady et al. 1992 (11).

TABLE 8-5. **Potential risks and benefits of hormone replacement therapy**

Outcome	Unopposed estrogen	Estrogen/progestin
Potential benefit		
Relief of vasomotor symptoms	Yes	Yes
Relief of urinary symptoms, vaginal dryness	Yes	Yes
Reduction of risk of cardio-vascular disease	Risk reduction of about 35%.	May also reduce risk; data not sufficient to estimate magnitude of risk reduction.
Reduction of risk of osteoporosis	Risk reduction of hip fractures about 25%; of vertebral fractures at least 50%.	Probably protects against fractures, but data still limited.
Increased life expectancy	By reduction of lifetime probability of coronary heart disease and osteoporosis, life expectancy generally increased.	Life expectancy probably increased, though possibly not as much as with unopposed estrogen. In women at high risk for breast cancer, life expectancy may actually be decreased.

Potential risk		
Endometrial cancer	Risk increases with duration of estrogen use; is about eightfold for 10–20 years of use. Risk of death probably not as high, because endometrial cancer is generally curable, especially in estrogen users.	Risk not increased.
Breast cancer	Controversial. Risk probably not increased among women who take estrogen for a short time (less than 5 years). Risk may increase somewhat (about 25%) if estrogen taken long term (10–20 years).	Controversial. May be a 25% risk increase with long-term use; there is concern that risk could be somewhat higher.
Side effects and vaginal bleeding	Bloating, headache, breast tenderness—usually mild (5%–10% of women taking estrogen). Side effects often improve after a few months. In women with a uterus, unpredictable uterine bleeding (35%–40% of treated women per year).	Bloating, weight gain, irritability, depression—usually mild—dose-dependent. Unpredictable endometrial bleeding (30%–50% of women during first 6–8 months of treatment), usually light and transient.

Source. Adapted in part from American College of Physicians 1992 (14).

risk for breast cancer, hormone replacement should be undertaken with careful considerations of these potential risks and benefits (Table 8–5).

As with oral contraceptives, certain preparations and dosages of hormones are better tolerated than others. For the 5%–10% of women who have difficulties with side effects, dosages and preparations may be adjusted to minimize side effects. In some women, estrogen may cause mild breast tenderness, bloating, and headache. Side effects that have been associated with progestin include bloating, weight gain, irritability, and dysphoria (11, 13).

Some studies suggest that estrogen may have a mood-enhancing effect in postmenopausal women, particularly in surgically menopausal women (14). However, estrogen alone does not appear to be effective in the treatment of clinical depression in perimenopausal or postmenopausal women.

■ EVALUATION AND TREATMENT OF DEPRESSION

The psychiatric evaluation of the middle-aged depressed woman should include an assessment of menstrual cycle patterns, vasomotor symptoms, and sexual function. Because a woman may not be aware of vasomotor symptoms occurring at night, it is important to ask if her nightclothes or sheets are damp or wet when she wakes up. Sleep disruption in middle-aged women is often the result of nighttime hot flashes and night sweats.

Hormonal evaluation on day 2 or 3 of the menstrual cycle may reveal elevated FSH and depressed estradiol levels. Thyroid function should also be evaluated, because women over 40 are at particular risk for thyroid disorders, and hypothyroidism may contribute to depressive symptoms. The patient should be referred for a full medical examination to rule out health problems (e.g., autoimmune disorders, endocrine disor-

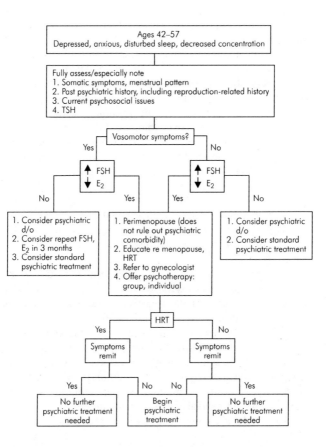

FIGURE 8–1. **Psychiatric evaluation of the middle-aged depressed woman: special considerations.**
Note. TSH = thyroid-stimulating hormone; FSH = follicle-stimulating hormone; d/o = disorder; E₂ = estradiol; HRT = hormone replacement therapy.

ders, heart disease, cancer) that may contribute to depressed mood.

If a perimenopausal woman is experiencing mild to moderate depressed mood, irritability, insomnia, and poor concentration in association with frequent or distressing hot flashes or night sweats, a trial of hormone replacement therapy may relieve both the vasomotor and the psychological symptoms.

However, if her depressive symptoms do not improve within 1–2 weeks, she should be offered standard psychiatric treatment, including psychotherapy and antidepressant medications. Treatment of the perimenopausal woman who meets criteria for a major depressive episode involves the usual psychiatric treatment modalities, including psychotherapy and pharmacotherapy. Estrogen replacement therapy, although useful for vasomotor symptoms and long-term postmenopausal medical complications, is not sufficient to treat a major depressive episode (Figure 8–1).

Because depressive symptoms in the perimenopausal years may be associated with psychosocial stressors, these stressors should be addressed in the treatment. The perimenopausal woman should be encouraged to discuss other sources of stress, including possible interpersonal stress, changing sexuality on her part or that of her partner, new-onset health problems, shifting role expectations, and new responsibilities, such as caring for aging and ill parents. In addition to individual psychotherapy, referrals to caregiver support groups, assistance with obtaining financial support, and attention to chronic medical problems are important aspects of the treatment.

■ REFERENCES

1. American Psychiatric Association: Diagnostic and Statistical Manual: Mental Disorders. Washington, DC, American Psychiatric Association, 1952
2. American Psychiatric Association: Diagnostic and Statistical Man-

ual of Mental Disorders, 2nd Edition. Washington, DC, American Psychiatric Association, 1968

3. American Psychiatric Association: Diagnostic and Statistical Manual of Mental Disorders, 3rd Edition. Washington, DC, American Psychiatric Association, 1980

4. Kaufert PA, Gilbert P, Tate R: The Manitoba Project: a reexamination of the link between menopause and depression. Maturitas 14:143–155, 1992

5. Matthews KA, Wing RA, Kuller LH: Influences of natural menopause on psychological characteristics and symptoms of middle-aged healthy women. J Consult Clin Psychol 58:345–351, 1990

6. Stewart DE, Boydell KM: Psychological distress during menopause: association across the reproductive life cycle. Int J Psychiatry Med 23:157–162, 1993

7. Avis NE, McKinlay SM: A longitudinal analysis of women's attitudes towards menopause: results from the Massachusetts Women's Health Study. Maturitas 13:65–79, 1991

8. Avis NE, McKinlay SM: The Massachusetts Women's Health Study: an epidemiologic investigation of the menopause. JAMWA 50:45–49, 1995

9. Stone AB, Pearlstein TB: Evaluation and treatment of changes in mood, sleep and sexual functioning associated with menopause. Obstet Gynecol Clin North Am 1:391–403, 1994

10. Sherwin BB, Gelfand MM, Brender W: Androgen enhances sexual motivation in females: a prospective, crossover study of sex steroid administration in the surgical menopause. Psychosom Med 47:339–351, 1985

11. Grady D, Rubin SM, Petitti DB, et al: Hormone therapy to prevent disease and prolong life in postmenopausal women. Ann Intern Med 117:1016–1037, 1992

12. Belchetz PE: Hormonal treatment of postmenopausal women. N Engl J Med 330:1062–1071, 1994

13. American College of Physicians: Guidelines for counseling postmenopausal women about preventive hormone therapy. Ann Intern Med 117:1038–1041, 1992

14. Sherwin BB: Affective changes with estrogen and androgen replacement therapy in surgically menopausal women. J Affect Disord 14:177–187, 1988

GENDER ISSUES IN THE TREATMENT OF MAJOR MENTAL ILLNESS

■ SCHIZOPHRENIA IN WOMEN

Epidemiology

Significant gender differences exist in the course and manifestation of schizophrenia. Although the incidence of schizophrenia appears to be approximately equal in men and women, the onset tends to occur later in women. In men, rates of new-onset schizophrenia reach a peak between ages 15 and 24. For women, the peak occurs between ages 20 and 29. About 15% of schizophrenic women do not develop the illness until their mid- or late 40s (1) (see Table 9–1). For men, onset of the illness after age 40 is rare.

Other gender differences include a more favorable premorbid history in women, including fewer premorbid abnormalities of personality (e.g., schizoid traits) and better premorbid social and occupational functioning (1). Women with schizophrenia tend to have more affective and positive symptoms than men and fewer negative symptoms, such as social withdrawal and lack of drive. Structural brain abnormalities, such as increased ventricle size and decreased hippocampal volume, appear to be less common in women patients with schizophrenia (2). Be-

9

TABLE 9–1.   **Gender differences in schizophrenia**

Compared to men, women

  Are less likely to have structural brain abnormalities

  Are more likely to have relatives with the illness

  Are more likely to have late-onset schizophrenia

  Are less likely to have comorbid substance abuse

  Are less likely to commit suicide

  Tend to exhibit more positive and fewer negative symptoms

  Tend to exhibit more affective symptoms

  Tend to respond to lower doses of neuroleptics

  Maintain better social functioning (e.g., higher rate of
     employment, marriage)

---

cause relatives of women with schizophrenia are more likely
than relatives of men to develop the illness, some researchers
have suggested that schizophrenia is a more heritable illness in
women and that environmental factors, such as birth complications, may be of more etiological significance in men (2).

Special Considerations in Treatment

Issues in the treatment of women with schizophrenia are listed
in Table 9–2.

  Compared to men, women respond better to treatment and
usually require lower doses of medication. The more favorable
treatment response and course of illness in women have led to
speculation that estrogen may have a protective effect against
schizophrenia (3). Animal studies show that estrogen has antidopaminergic (i.e., neuroleptic-like) activity and may therefore
protect women against psychosis. Notably, symptomatic exacerbation of schizophrenia has been observed during the
low-estrogen phases of the menstrual cycle (3, 4) and in perimenopausal years (5).

  Because schizophrenic women on neuroleptic medication

TABLE 9–2. **Special issues in treating women with schizophrenia**

Assess for possible symptomatic variation across the menstrual cycle

Inquire about menstrual irregularities, amenorrhea, galactorrhea; measure serum prolactin levels

Counsel about avoiding unwanted sexual advances

Counsel about birth control

Inquire about recent unprotected intercourse; consider obtaining pregnancy test

have high rates of menstrual irregularities and amenorrhea, menstrual-cycle patterns should be assessed. For women of childbearing age with menstrual cycle disturbances, a β-human chorionic gonadotropin (β-HCG) level should be obtained to test for pregnancy. Other relatively common causes of menstrual cycle irregularity include hypothyroidism and primary hyperprolactinemia. However, the most likely cause of menstrual irregularity in schizophrenic women is the use of neuroleptic medication. Neuroleptics increase levels of the pituitary hormone prolactin, which in turn inhibits estrogen release. Because estrogen is necessary for maturation of the ovarian follicles, a hypoestrogenic state can prevent ovulation and produce amenorrhea. Amenorrhea is not unusual when prolactin levels are greater than 60 ng/mL (normal prolactin levels = 5–25 ng/mL) (6). Galactorrhea, or nipple discharge, may also occur with elevated prolactin levels. If prolactin levels exceed 100 ng/mL, a brain-imaging study (preferably magnetic resonance imaging [MRI]), should be obtained to assess the likelihood of a prolactin-secreting pituitary tumor. Additional causes of elevated prolactin include pregnancy, nursing, stress, weight loss, opiate use, and oral contraceptives (7).

If hyperprolactinemia is determined to be secondary to the use of a neuroleptic, the dose should be tapered whenever possible. Alternatively, bromocriptine at 2.5–7.5 mg bid reduces prolactin levels. Although bromocriptine is a dopamine agonist, it does not appear to exacerbate psychosis at this dosage. To minimize nausea, a common side effect, bromocriptine should be taken with food. A third strategy is initiation of an oral contraceptive. This approach returns the patient to regular menstrual cycling and, by restoring estrogen, protects against the long-term adverse effects of a hypoestrogenic state, such as osteoporosis and heart disease. Additionally, it has the advantage of providing contraception. Prolactin levels, however, may rise with use of oral contraceptives and thus should be monitored closely. If prolactin levels rise or amenorrhea persists, the woman should be referred for a gynecological and endocrinological evaluation.

Schizophrenic women are at particular risk for pregnancy because of ineffective use of birth control and high rates of sexual assault. Even women with neuroleptic-induced amenorrhea may occasionally ovulate and thus can become pregnant. Teaching women patients about birth control and about strategies to avoid unwanted sexual advances are important aspects of treatment.

■ DEPRESSION IN WOMEN

Epidemiology

A number of large epidemiological studies have consistently found that women are more likely than men to suffer from depressive disorders (8–12). The Epidemiologic Catchment Area Study, the largest survey of psychiatric disorders in North America, reported a female-to-male ratio of 1.96:1, with a lifetime prevalence of mood disorders of 10.2% in women and 5.2% in men (13). Using a structured psychiatric interview to evaluate a representative sample of the general population, the National Comorbidity Survey (Table 9–3) reported higher rates

TABLE 9–3. National Comorbidity Survey rates of affective disorders in men and women

Affective disorder	Men (%)		Women (%)		Total (%)	
	Lifetime	12 months	Lifetime	12 months	Lifetime	12 months
Major depressive episode	12.7	7.7	21.3	12.9	17.1	10.3
Manic episode	1.6	1.4	1.7	1.3	1.6	1.3
Dysthymia	4.8	2.1	8.0	3.0	6.4	2.5
Any affective disorder	14.7	8.5	23.9	14.1	19.3	11.3

Source.   Data extracted from Kessler et al. 1993 (12).

of depression in both sexes, with a lifetime rate of depression of 21.3% in women and 12.7% in men (11, 12), producing a female-to-male ratio of 1.68:1 (11, 12). The increased prevalence of depression in women begins in adolescence and is a cross-cultural phenomenon (14–17). For dysthymia, the prevalence is twice as high in women, with lifetime rates of 5.4% for women and 2.6% for men (17). The preponderance of women is even higher for atypical depression (i.e., depression characterized by mood reactivity and at least one of the following: hypersomnia, hyperphagia, leaden paralysis, rejection sensitivity) and seasonal affective disorder (SAD) (18).

Special Considerations in Treatment

In providing pharmacological treatment to women of reproductive age, it is important to keep in mind the possibility of pregnancy. Thus, sexually active women should be advised to use an effective method of contraception. For women who are planning to conceive and who may require continued use of medication during pregnancy, choosing an antidepressant that appears safe during pregnancy may avoid the need to switch medications following conception.

Some women who suffer from depression experience premenstrual exacerbation of their symptoms (19) and thus may exhibit premenstrual symptom worsening despite successful treatment of depression at other times of the month (see Chapter 2). For women who exhibit monthly exacerbation of a depression that is otherwise responsive to pharmacotherapy, it may be useful to chart the timing of the symptoms. If there appears to be a consistent premenstrual exacerbation of depression, an increase in antidepressant dose 7–10 days before onset of menses may help maintain euthymia throughout the cycle (20).

SAD is 4–6 times more prevalent in women than men (18). Light therapy (2,500-lux light box for 1–2 hours per day) or an antidepressant during the symptomatic period may be effective strategies.

Through their serotonergic activity, antidepressants (both the tricyclic antidepressants and the selective serotonin reuptake inhibitors) may cause hyperprolactinemia (21). Although this effect occurs much less frequently with antidepressants than with neuroleptics, it is important to keep it in mind, particularly for patients who complain of amenorrhea, galactorrhea, or breast pain. Women are far more likely than men to have eating disorders, and many women with eating disorders experience comorbid depression. Because patients with anorexia or bulimia may have electrolyte imbalances that put them at particular risk for seizures, medications that reduce the seizure threshold (bupropion, clomipramine, maprotiline) should be avoided.

Women are at risk for depression during the first 6 postpartum months (see Chapter 4), and this is particularly true for women with histories of depression and postpartum depression. For many of these women, prophylaxis with an antidepressant may be essential for preventing a recurrent episode (22). Some data show that women with histories of depression related to the use of oral contraceptives, the premenstruum, or the postpartum are at risk of perimenopausal depression (23). Particularly in women with histories of depression, longitudinal monitoring for recurrence of depression at vulnerable points in the female life cycle may allow for the rapid implementation of treatment and the prevention of a relapse.

■ BIPOLAR DISORDER IN WOMEN

Epidemiology

Although bipolar disorder occurs equally in men and women, there are significant gender differences in its course and manifestation (Table 9–4). Women with the disorder appear to experience more depressions than do men with the disorder, whereas men experience more manic episodes. In addition, dysphoric (mixed) mania may be more common in women (24).

Women with bipolar disorder are approximately three times as likely as men to experience rapid cycling, defined as four or more affective episodes per year (24, 25). Why rapid cycling should occur more often in women is unclear; one possibility is that, because women with bipolar disorder experience more depressions than men, they are more likely to take antidepressants, which may precipitate rapid cycling (26). Additionally, thyroid dysfunction is more common in women, and hypothyroidism has been implicated in rapid cycling. Of note, the data on thyroid function and rapid cycling are mixed, as are data on the use of thyroid supplementation for treatment of rapid cycling.

Women with bipolar disorder may experience premenstrual relapse or exacerbation of symptoms (49). Mood fluctuations in women with rapid-cycling bipolar disorder, however, do not appear to vary consistently with the menstrual cycle (24, 27). These women should be encouraged to chart their moods daily, so that the relationship between menstrual cycle phases and mood changes can be addressed. For women whose mood consistently deteriorates premenstrually, it is helpful to obtain blood levels of medication both premenstrually and in the week postmenses, as there are reports of fluctuating plasma level of mood stabilizers across the menstrual cycle (49).

TABLE 9–4. **Gender differences in bipolar disorder**

As compared to men, women

    Are more likely to be rapid cyclers

    Are more likely to develop lithium-induced hypothyroidism

    Experience more depressions

    May experience more dysphoric manias

Special Considerations in Treatment

Special issues in the treatment of women with bipolar disorder are listed in Table 9–5.

Because women taking lithium are at significant risk of developing lithium-induced hypothyroidism, thyroid function should be monitored at least every 6 months. Women older than 40 are particularly at risk for thyroid dysfunction, whether lithium induced or from other etiologies.

By inducing hormone clearance and metabolism, carbamazepine may reduce the efficacy of oral contraceptives. Women with bipolar disorder who are taking carbamazepine and oral contraceptives should therefore be advised to use a different or an additional form of contraception. Postmenopausal women taking carbamazepine may find that they need higher doses of hormone replacement to reduce hypoestrogenemia-induced vasomotor symptoms (hot flashes, night sweats).

In a single small preliminary study, valproic acid has been associated with increased rates of menstrual disturbances, hyperandrogenism, and polycystic ovaries, especially in women

---

TABLE 9–5. **Special concerns in treating women with bipolar disorder**

Symptoms may recur or worsen premenstrually.

Medication levels may fluctuate across the menstrual cycle.

Carbamazepine may render oral contraceptives ineffective through its induction of liver enzymes.

Psychotropic agents (e.g., neuroleptics and valproic acid) may produce menstrual cycle disturbances).

Mood-stabilizing medications, especially valproic acid and carbamazepine, are associated with relatively high rates of fetal anomalies when used during the first trimester of pregnancy (see Chapter 4).

Women with bipolar disorder are at significant risk for postpartum psychosis (see Chapter 5).

---

under age 20 (28). Neuroleptics, sometimes used in the treatment of acute mania, may cause amenorrhea or menstrual disturbances by elevation of serum prolactin levels.

A menstrual history is essential for assessing patterns of bipolar-disorder symptom exacerbation in relation to the menstrual cycle and for monitoring psychotropic-induced disturbances of the menstrual cycle pattern.

■ ANXIETY DISORDERS IN WOMEN

Epidemiology

Anxiety disorders are the most prevalent of psychiatric disorders, affecting 1 in 10 people in the United States (14, 29). As a class, anxiety disorders are more prevalent in women than in men, and women with anxiety disorders are more likely than men to experience comorbid depression (30, 31). Panic with agoraphobia is two to three times more common in women, and generalized anxiety disorder and posttraumatic stress disorder are twice as frequent in women (29, 32, 33). Alcoholic women are more likely to have panic disorder with agoraphobia than are alcoholic men (34). Whether agoraphobia is a precipitant for alcoholism in women is unclear. Although the prevalence rates for obsessive-compulsive disorder (OCD) are approximately equal for men and women, women appear to have an earlier onset than men (25 years in women versus 20 years in men) (35).

In a cross-national survey of drug use among men and women, the rate of anxiolytic drug use in women was double that of men (36). Anxiety in women is a major reason for the increased use of anxiolytics and other psychotropic medications in women (37).

The reasons for the preponderance of anxiety disorders in women are not clear. A recent large epidemiological study of female twins found that, although generalized anxiety disorder is moderately familial, environmental experiences play an important role in determining which individuals will be affected (38). Similarly, only modest heritability (30%) has been demonstrated for panic disorder, and epidemiological research has failed to separate genetic and environmental factors as etiological in the transmission of panic disorder (39).

Other possible causes for the preponderance of anxiety disorders in women include the increased demands of work and family placed on today's women, reproduction-related alterations in hormones, less encouragement of self-sufficiency and self-confidence in girls than in boys, and histories of physical and sexual abuse (40).

Special Considerations in Treatment

Evaluation for anxiety should first rule out medical conditions that present with anxious symptoms. In evaluating women patients for anxiety, the clinician should give particular attention to certain medical disorders. Complaints of chest discomfort, diaphoresis, and tachycardia warrant a thorough diagnostic evaluation for heart disease. Women with these symptoms are more likely than men to be misdiagnosed as having an anxiety disorder and less likely than men to receive a cardiac workup (41). Postmenopausal women with family histories of cardiovascular disease, especially if they are not on hormone replacement, are at particular risk.

Patients with hypo- or hyperthyroidism may develop panic attacks with the onset of their thyroid condition. A thyroid panel should thus be obtained in women reporting tachycardia, anxiety, diaphoresis, temperature intolerance, or tremor. Thyroid disease is more prevalent in women than in men, particularly women older than 40. Other medical illnesses that affect women more than men and that may present with symptoms of anxiety include systemic lupus erythematosus and iron deficiency anemia.

Nicotine and caffeine use should be assessed in women reporting symptoms of anxiety and insomnia. Whereas the rate of cigarette smoking in the general population is declining, the rate in teenage girls and women has experienced a particularly steep rise.

A full assessment of a patient's medications should be part of the workup for an anxiety disorder. A number of medications may induce symptoms of anxiety, including nonsteroidal anti-inflammatory agents, decongestants, steroids, and appetite-suppressant medications.

Perimenopausal women may experience heat sensations, sweating, shortness of breath, and anxiety. For these women, vasomotor symptoms may be mistaken for panic or anxiety attacks (see Chapter 8). A history of menstrual cycle alterations and a follicle-stimulating hormone (FSH) level and an estradiol level on day 2 or day 3 of the menstrual cycle (for women who are still cycling) can identify perimenopausal status. Hormone replacement, rather than anxiolytic or antidepressant medication, may suffice to resolve these symptoms if they are of vasomotor origin.

Although women and men appear to have an equal prevalence of OCD, women seem to have more obsessions related to food and weight than do men, and women are also more likely to suffer from comorbid anorexia (42). It is therefore important to evaluate carefully all women with OCD for symptoms of restrictive-eating disorders.

■ ALCOHOL AND SUBSTANCE ABUSE IN WOMEN

Alcoholism

Women are significantly less likely than men to have a drinking problem. The prevalence rate of alcoholism in men has been estimated at more than twice that in women (43). Nevertheless, alcoholism in adult women is not uncommon; it is estimated at

6% (44). Rates of alcoholism in young women, whose drinking patterns are approaching those of men, may be even higher (43).

Gender-specific physiological differences cause women to be more intoxicated than men when they drink an equal amount of alcohol per unit of body weight. Some reports suggest that alcohol dehydrogenase, the enzyme that degrades alcohol, is significantly less active in women (43). In addition, because women have more body fat and less body water than men, they reach higher blood alcohol levels, because alcohol is diluted in total body water. Thus, although heavy drinking is considered more than four drinks a day in men, it may be as little as one and one-half drinks a day for women (44). Alcohol-related medical complications (e.g., peptic ulcer, liver disease, anemia, cerebral atrophy) develop more quickly in women, and women have higher relative mortality rates from alcoholism than do men (43).

Risk factors for alcoholism.   Risk factors in women include a personal history of sexual abuse, a family history of substance abuse, and adult antisocial personality disorder (Table 9–6). Depression is a much more significant risk factor for alcohol abuse in women than in men (43). In fact, depression tends to precede alcoholism in women, whereas in men it tends to follow alcoholism (43). Living with a substance-abusing partner is also a major risk factor for women, and it can reduce the likelihood that treatment will be successful.

TABLE 9–6.   **Risk factors for alcoholism in women**

History of sexual abuse

Clinical depression

Living with a substance-abusing partner

Family history of alcoholism

Antisocial personality disorder

Drug Abuse

As with alcohol abuse, the rates of abuse of hallucinogens and opiates are higher in men than in women. Cocaine and amphetamine abuse, however, are equally prevalent in men and women. Compared with men, women are less likely to be cocaine injectors and more likely to be cocaine smokers and sniffers (45). Women may be motivated to use stimulants for weight control purposes. Rates of prescription drug abuse are higher in women, possibly because women go to doctors more often than men. Also, women substance abusers are more likely to have comorbid psychiatric diagnoses than men and thus to receive prescription medications (e.g., sedatives).

Risk factors for drug abuse include a family history of drug abuse, adult antisocial personality disorder, depression, and involvement with a drug-dependent partner (46).

Screening and treatment. Special considerations in the screening and treatment of substance-abusing women are listed in Table 9–7. Any woman who presents with complaints of depression, anxiety, insomnia, sexual dysfunction, job problems, or family and marital conflicts should be assessed for substance abuse. Of particular concern is the direct request for specific prescription medications. Women who report great preoccupation with their weight should be assessed for the use of diet pills or stimulants. Although a careful history is the most important part of the evaluation, the CAGE questionnaire (Table 9–8) is a helpful screening instrument for alcoholism. Laboratory values are not reliably useful to screen for alcoholism, but they can help confirm the diagnosis. Elevated results on liver function tests, primarily γ-glutamyltransferase (GGT), and a high mean corpuscular volume (MCV) suggest a history of extensive drinking. Medical problems such as peptic ulcer, hypertension, anemia, and liver disease result from heavy alcohol consumption and should prompt investigation into drinking patterns.

TABLE 9–7. **Special issues for substance-abusing women**

Comorbid depressive and anxiety disorders are common.

Premenstrual tension may exacerbate substance abuse.

The dosage of alcohol that produces intoxication is lower in women than in men, even after controlling for body weight.

Medical consequences of alcoholism progress faster in women than in men.

Child care concerns may prevent a woman from obtaining treatment.

Stigmatizing by society may inhibit a woman from admitting her alcohol or substance abuse.

Excessive preoccupation with weight control may lead to stimulant abuse.

TABLE 9–8. **CAGE questionnaire**

Have you ever felt you ought to **C**ut down on your drinking?

Have people **A**nnoyed you by criticizing your drinking?

Have you ever felt bad or **G**uilty about your drinking?

Have you ever had a drink first thing in the morning to steady your nerves or get rid of a hangover (**E**ye-opener)?

Note. CAGE = **C**ut [down], **A**nnoyed, **G**uilty, **E**ye-opener.
Source. Adapted from Ewing 1984 (48).

Alcohol- and drug-related legal and employment problems are helpful in making a diagnosis of substance abuse, although more so in men than in women. Women, on the other hand, are more likely to have substance-abuse–related family, interpersonal, and health problems (47). Because depression frequently precedes or is comorbid with substance abuse in women, all women alcoholics should be assessed for current and previous depressive episodes. If a woman has a history of depression preceding her substance dependence, she is at risk for a depressive relapse as she recovers (43, 46). Treatment of depression may decrease the likelihood that the patient will return to substance use. For the same reason, comorbid anxiety disorders should be treated. Addictive prescription medications are best avoided, because women with alcoholism are at risk for prescription drug abuse. An assessment for premenstrual symptoms is important, because up to two-thirds of alcoholic women may drink to self-medicate premenstrual tension (49). Treatment of the premenstrual symptoms may reduce the alcohol use.

For any treatment plan to be effective, it is essential for the substance-abusing woman to accept that she has an illness and to recognize the interpersonal, psychological, and medical consequences of her drug use. Referrals to self-help groups—including Alcoholics Anonymous, Cocaine Anonymous, and Women for Sobriety, an all-woman support group—are important aspects of treatment. The woman's family should be involved; family support and concern may help motivate the patient to remain in recovery. Family members can benefit from referrals to Al-Anon. Because a woman's drinking or drug use pattern is greatly influenced by that of her partner, her likelihood of reaching sobriety is enhanced if her partner is sober. Thus, an evaluation of the partner's drinking or drug use patterns is important. If the partner also has a substance use problem, he or she should be encouraged to obtain treatment. Family and marital conflicts may contribute to a woman's drinking or drug use and should be explored. Attention should be given to child care needs that may interfere with a woman's ability to obtain treatment.

Societal stigmatization of women drinkers may cause women to hide drinking problems. Women may also fear losing custody of their children if they reveal their alcoholism. It is therefore essential that women alcoholics be treated in a nonjudgmental and supportive manner. Group and individual therapy are helpful, particularly in addressing issues of shame and low self-esteem and in promoting assertiveness.

■ REFERENCES

1. Goldstein JM, Link BG: Gender and the expression of schizophrenia. J Psychiatr Res 22:141–155, 1988
2. Castle DJ, Murray RM: The neurodevelopmental basis of sex differences in schizophrenia. Psychol Med 21:565–575, 1991
3. Szymanski S, Lieberman JA, Alvir JM, et al: Gender differences in onset of illness, treatment response, course, and biologic indexes in first-episode schizophrenic patients. Am J Psychiatry 152:698–703, 1995
4. Seeman MV, Lang M: The role of estrogens in schizophrenia gender differences. Schizophr Bull 16:185–194, 1990
5. Seeman MV: Current outcome in schizophrenia: women vs men. Acta Psychiatr Scand 73:609–617, 1986
6. Seeman MV: Interaction of sex, age, and neuroleptic dose. Compr Psychiatry 24:125–128, 1983
7. Marken PA, Radwan FH, Fisher JN: Management of psychotropic-induced hyperprolactinemia. Clin Pharm 11:851–856, 1992
8. Weissman MM, Klerman GL: Sex differences and the epidemiology of depression. Arch Gen Psychiatry 34:98–111, 1977
9. Boyd JH, Weissman MM: Epidemiology of affective disorders: a reexamination and future directions. Arch Gen Psychiatry 38:1039–1046, 1981
10. Weissman MM, Leaf PJ, Holzer CE III, et al: The epidemiology of depression: an update on sex differences in rates. J Affect Disord 7:179–188, 1984
11. Kessler RC, McGonagle KA, Zhao S, et al: Lifetime and 12-month prevalence of DSM-III-R psychiatric disorders in the United States: results from the National Comorbidity Survey. Arch Gen Psychiatry 51:8–19, 1994
12. Kessler RC, McGonagle KA, Swartz M, et al: Sex and depression in the National Comorbidity Survey, I: lifetime prevalence, chronicity and recurrence. J Affect Disord 29:85–96, 1993
13. Weissman MM, Livingston Mb, Leaf PJ, et al: Affective disorders, in Psychiatric Disorders in America. Edited by Robins LN, Regier DA. New York, Free Press, 1991, p 53
14. Bland RC, Orn R, Newman SC: Lifetime prevalence of psychiatric disorders in Edmonton. Acta Psychiatr Scand 77 (suppl 338):24–32, 1988

15. Wells JE, Bushnell JA, Hornblow AR, et al: Christchurch psychiatric epidemiology study, I: methodology and lifetime prevalence for specific psychiatric disorders. Aust N Z J Psychiatry 23: 315–326, 1989

16. Wittchen HU, Essau GC, Von Zerssen D, et al: Lifetime and six-month prevalence of mental disorders in the Munich Follow-up Study. Eur Arch Psychiatry Clin Neurosci 241:247–258, 1992

17. Weissman MM, Bland R, Joyce PR, et al: Sex differences in rates of depression: cross-national perspectives. J Affect Disord 29:77–84, 1993

18. Rosenthal NE, Sack DA, Gillin JC, et al: Seasonal affective disorder: a description of the syndrome and preliminary findings with light therapy. Arch Gen Psychiatry 41:72–80, 1984

19. Yonkers KA, White K: Premenstrual exacerbation of depression: one process or two? J Clin Psychiatry 53:289–292, 1992

20. Jensvold MF, Reed K, Jarrett DB, et al: Menstrual cycle- related depressive symptoms treated with variable antidepressant dosage. Journal of Women's Health 1:109–115, 1992

21. Marken PA, Haykal RF, Fisher JN: Management of psychotropic-induced hyperprolactinemia. Clin Pharm 11:831–836, 1991

22. Wisner KL, Wheeler SB: Prevention of recurrent postpartum major depression. Hosp Community Psychiatry 45:1191–1196, 1994

23. Stewart DE, Boydell KM: Psychological distress during menopause: association across the reproductive life cycle. Int J Psychiatry Med 23:157–162, 1993

24. Liebenluft E: Women with bipolar illness: clinical and research issues. Am J Psychiatry 153:163–173, 1996

25. Alarcon RD: Rapid cycling affective disorders: a clinical review. Compr Psychiatry 26:522–540, 1985

26. Wehr TA, Goodwin FK: Rapid cycling in manic depressives induced by tricyclic antidepressants. Arch Gen Psychiatry 36:555–559, 1979

27. Wehr TA, Sack DA, Rosenthal NE, et al: Rapid cycling affective disorder: contributing factors and treatment responses in 51 patients. Am J Psychiatry 145:179–184, 1988

28. Isojarvi JIT, Laatikainen TJ, Pakarinen AJ, et al: Polycystic ovaries and hyperandrogenism in women taking valproate for epilepsy. N Engl J Med 329:1383–1388, 1993

29. Robins LN, Helzer JE, Weissman MM, et al: Lifetime prevalence

of specific disorders in three sites. Arch Gen Psychiatry 41:949–958, 1984

30. Pajer K: New strategies in the treatment of depression in women. J Clin Psychiatry 56 (suppl 2):30–37, 1995

31. Scheibe G, Albus M: Age at onset, precipitating events, sex distribution, and co-occurrence of anxiety disorders. Psychopathology 25:11–18, 1992

32. Bourdon KH, Boyd JH, Rae DS, et al: Gender differences in phobias: results of the ECA community survey. Journal of Anxiety Disorders 2:227–241, 1988

33. Schneier FR, Johnson J, Hornig CD, et al: Social phobia: comorbidity and morbidity in an epidemiologic sample. Arch Gen Psychiatry 49:282–288, 1992

34. Task Force on Panic Anxiety and Its Treatments: Panic anxiety and panic disorder, in Panic Anxiety and Its Treatments. Edited by Klerman GL, Hirschfield RMA, Weissman MM, et al. Washington, DC, American Psychiatric Press, 1993, pp 3–38

35. Flament MF, Rapoport JL: Childhood obsessive-compulsive disorder, in New Findings in Obsessive-Compulsive Disorder. Edited by Insel TR. Washington, DC, American Psychiatric Press, 1984, pp 23–43

36. Balter MB, Levine L, Manheimer DI: Cross-national study of the extent of anti-anxiety/sedative drug use. N Engl J Med 290:769–774, 1974

37. Baum C, Kennedy DL, Forbes MB, et al: Drug use in the United States in 1981. JAMA 251:1293–1297, 1984

38. Kendler KS, Neale MC, Kessler RC, et al: Panic disorder in women: a population-based twin study. Psychol Med 23:397–406, 1993

39. Kendler KS, Neale MC, Kessler RC, et al: Generalized anxiety disorder in women: a population-based twin study. Arch Gen Psychiatry 49:267–272, 1992

40. Zerbe KJ: Anxiety disorders in women. Bull Menninger Clin 59 (suppl A):A38–A52, 1995

41. Wenger NK, Speroff L, Packard B: Cardiovascular health and disease in women. N Engl J Med 329:247–256, 1993

42. Kasvikis JG, Tsakiris F, Marks IM: Women with obsessive-compulsive disorder frequently report a past history of anorexia nervosa. International Journal of Eating Disorders 5:1069–1075, 1986

43. Blume SB: Gender differences in alcohol-related disorders. Harvard Review of Psychiatry 2:7–14, 1994

44. Cyr MG, Moulton AW: Substance abuse in women. Obstet Gynecol Clin North Am 17:905–925, 1990

45. Gossop M, Griffiths P, Powis B, et al: Cocaine: patterns of use, route of administration, and severity of dependence. Br J Psychiatry 164:660–664, 1994

46. Griffin ML, Weiss RD, Mirin SM, et al: Comparison of male and female cocaine abusers. Arch Gen Psychiatry 46:122–126, 1989

47. Cyr MG, Moulton AW: The physician's role in prevention, detection, and treatment of alcohol abuse in women. Psychiatric Annals 23:454–462, 1993

48. Ewing JA: Detecting alcoholism: the CAGE questionnaire. JAMA 252:1905–1907, 1984

49. Hendrick V, Altshuler LL, Burt VK: Course of psychiatric disorders across the menstrual cycle. Harvard Review of Psychiatry 4:200–207, 1996

10

FEMALE-SPECIFIC CANCERS

■ BREAST CANCER

One in nine women will have breast cancer in her lifetime (1), making it the most prevalent of all cancers in women. The disease is rare in women under 30, rises among women in their early 40s, stabilizes, then increases again in women older than 55. Two-thirds of all breast cancer patients are older than 50. Women with certain risk factors (see Table 10–1), particularly a first-degree relative with breast cancer, tend to feel even more anxious about their likelihood of developing the disease.

The stress of being diagnosed with and treated for breast cancer is compounded by the worry of disfigurement. In the past decade, however, breast-sparing procedures have increasingly replaced radical mastectomies, dramatically reducing the effect on a woman's physical appearance following surgery. Although breast-conserving surgery has a beneficial effect on self-image and self-esteem, women may feel greater uncertainty about their long-term survival (1). Current research, however, suggests that breast-sparing procedures have outcomes equally favorable to those of radical mastectomies (1).

The treatment strategies for breast cancer are surgery, radiation therapy, and chemotherapy. Surgical procedures include the following: Radical mastectomy includes removal of the breast, the chest muscles, and the underarm lymph nodes. A modified radical mastectomy removes the breast, the under-

TABLE 10–1. **Risk factors for breast cancer**

Family history, especially in first-degree female relatives

First pregnancy after age 30

Nulliparity

Early menarche

Late menopause

Increasing age

Caucasian race

Obesity

Higher socioeconomic status

History of benign breast disease

Previous carcinoma in one breast, especially in premenopausal
women

Nicotine use

Alcohol use

Use of exogenous hormones (controversial)

arm lymph nodes, and the lining over the chest muscles. Total
(simple) mastectomy removes only the breast. Partial (segmental) mastectomy removes the tumor and some surrounding
tissue. Lumpectomy removes only the breast lump; it is followed by radiation therapy. Radiation therapy may also be used
after segmental or total mastectomy, particularly if cancer has
been found in the lymph nodes.

Adjuvant chemotherapy sometimes follows the surgery and
usually employs cyclophosphamide, methotrexate, 5-fluoro-
uracil, and adriamycin. For women with estrogen-receptor–
positive tumors, hormonal therapy with tamoxifen may
be used. Newer, experimental treatment strategies include
high-dose chemotherapy with granulocyte-macrophage
colony-stimulating factor (GM-CSF) or granulocyte-colony-
stimulating factor (G-CSF) or with bone marrow transplanta-
tion. Following mastectomy, breast reconstruction is an option

that may significantly enhance a woman's sense of sexuality and self-esteem.

■ GYNECOLOGICAL CANCER

Gynecological cancers produce significant stress, not only because they are life-threatening, but also because they affect organs associated with reproduction, sexuality, and femininity. In order of frequency, gynecological cancers affect the cervix, endometrium, ovary, vagina, and vulva. Ovarian cancer, however, produces the greatest mortality rate. Surgical treatments for gynecological cancers include hysterectomy, or removal of the uterus; ovariectomy, or removal of the ovaries; vulvectomy, or excision of the external genitalia; and pelvic exenteration, a more radical surgical procedure involving removal of the bladder, vagina, uterus, and rectum. Chemotherapeutic agents may be initiated following surgery, and usually include vincristine, vinblastine, and interferon. Following pelvic exenteration or vulvectomy, construction of a neovagina helps restore some sexual function.

Sexual problems following treatment may result from the physical effects of surgery or pelvic irradiation. Psychological issues associated with the cancer may also influence a woman's sexuality. They include a fear of recurrence of cancer and a decreased sense of femininity from loss of the uterus or other pelvic organs. The partner's attitude toward a woman's diagnosis and treatment also affects her sexuality. The partner's sexual interest following the surgery helps maintain a woman's sexual functioning (2).

■ PSYCHIATRIC CONSULTATION

A psychiatric consultation may be requested for a woman undergoing treatment for breast or gynecological cancer. In addition to a standard psychiatric assessment, attention should be given to issues that are particularly relevant to this population: depression and anxiety, interpersonal issues, and common fears and concerns.

Depression and Anxiety

A patient's physicians and family may dismiss her depressive symptoms as normal reactions to an illness and may attribute physical problems (poor appetite, fatigue, loss of sexual desire) to the illness and its treatment rather than to a mood disorder. A careful psychiatric assessment is therefore necessary. Breast cancer patients at highest risk for depression are those with a history of depression, with advanced cancer, and with significant pain (3, 4). A woman's coping style also influences her emotional state during treatment: a sense of helplessness and fatalism, in contrast to a sense of control over events, produces greater psychological morbidity (5). Organic etiologies for mood disorders in cancer patients include the depressive side effects of steroids and some chemotherapeutic agents (Table 10–2).

Psychiatric treatment strategies include supportive therapy and cognitive approaches to reduce a patient's sense of helplessness. Education about the treatment can increase a woman's sense of control and of the predictability of the situation.

Antidepressant medications, by enhancing appetite and sleep, may be helpful not only for mood but also for a patient's physical condition. Tricyclic antidepressants (TCAs) have the additional advantage of reducing pain. On the other hand, less sedating antidepressants may be preferable for patients experiencing lethargy or undergoing radiation therapy, a procedure associated with significant fatigue. There is a case report of tamoxifen-associated reduction in serum TCA and metabolite levels (7). For antidepressant-treated patients on tamoxifen or other medications that interact with the cytochrome P-450

TABLE 10–2. **Anticancer drugs associated with psychiatric side effects**

Drug	Delirium	Depression	Anxiety	Psychosis
		Side effect		
cisplatin	x	-	-	-
cyclophosphamide	x	-	-	-
dacarbazine	-	-	x	-
hexamethylamine	x	x	-	-
methotrexate	x	-	-	-
5-fluorouracil	x	-	-	-
vincristine	x	x	-	x
vinblastine	x	x	x	-
interferon	x	x	-	-
corticosteroids	x	-	-	x
tamoxifen	x	-	-	x (1 report)

Note. Empty cells indicate that side effect is not present.
Sources. Derived from McCartney 1993 (2) and Ron et al. 1992 (6).

system, it may be useful to check serum levels of parent and metabolite compounds and to raise the dose when clinically indicated.

Anxiety may be treated with cognitive-behavioral strategies (e.g., guided imagery, progressive relaxation) and with low doses of anxiolytic medications. For patients with initial insomnia secondary to anxiety, short-acting benzodiazepines such as oxazepam or temazepam may be useful for several weeks. Low dosages of trazodone (e.g., 50–100 mg per night) may also be helpful.

Patients should be counseled regarding sleep hygiene and avoidance of caffeine and alcohol. Women with cancer who have a history of heavy alcohol use may increase their alcohol intake and risk alcohol abuse or dependence. These women should be encouraged to share their concerns and fears with nonjudgmental professional or lay persons (including Alcoholics Anonymous sponsors). These helping persons can assist the patient with the reality of cancer and adapting to the illness.

Interpersonal Issues

The diagnosis and treatment of breast or gynecological cancer may have a significant effect on the woman's marital or sexual relationship. A woman's sense of sexuality and femininity may be reduced following surgery, particularly if the surgery was extensive. The pain of past sexual traumas may be revived during gynecological cancer treatment. Induced menopause from radical hysterectomy often precipitates hot flashes, cold sweats, and disturbed sleep, which frequently cannot be treated with hormone replacement therapy because it is contraindicated for patients with certain kinds of breast or gynecological cancers. Continued sleep deprivation may escalate into depression, irritability, and anxiety.

A woman's partner may fear hurting the woman by resuming sexual activity or may want to avoid seeing her surgical scars, as reminders of her illness and mortality. It may be helpful for a partner to be involved in the treatment decisions and to help with dressings and other postsurgical care. Conjoint education and supportive therapy are often beneficial as the couple deals with interpersonal issues and the resumption of sexual activity. Special consideration should be given to couples with a history of conflict or poor communication, because they are at greater risk for poor adjustment.

The availability of other interpersonal supports should be explored. Psychological intervention with a patient's family may enhance a sense of family unity and support. The Reach to Recovery program provides peer counseling, matching women who have had surgery for breast cancer with women who are facing it. Group therapy, offered by hospital-based cancer centers and local branches of the American Cancer Society, provides both psychological and practical support for the patient and family (see Appendix). An important statistic is that 10-year survival rates are greater in women who participate in group therapy than in women who do not (8).

Common Fears and Concerns

It is natural for a patient to have concerns about disfigurement, recurrence, pain, and death. Anxiety about the diagnosis may result in a delay in obtaining appropriate care. A patient may worry about the welfare of her children while she is in the hospital or in the event of her death. The psychiatrist may be particularly helpful as a liaison with the oncology team to ensure that the patient obtains adequate management of pain and nausea and that she is informed about her treatment course, options, and prognosis. Negative psychiatric side effects of chemotherapy should be assessed and managed with the aid of psychiatric consultation and follow-up. Interventions addressing practical issues, such as child care and financial concerns, can significantly reduce a patient's anxiety while she undergoes treatment. The patient should also be reassured that all possible therapeutic measures have been employed, particularly if her cancer is terminal, because this information may help her accept the cancer.

■ REFERENCES

1. Rowland JH, Holland JC: Breast cancer, in Handbook of Psycho-oncology. Edited by Holland JC, Rowland JH. New York, Oxford University Press, 1989, pp 188–207
2. McCartney CF: Gynecologic oncology, in Psychological Aspects of Women's Health Care. Edited by Stewart DE, Stotland NL. Washington, DC, American Psychiatric Press, 1993, pp 291–312
3. Cain EN, Kohorn EI, Quinlan DM, et al: Psychosocial reactions to the diagnosis of gynecologic cancer. Obstet Gynecol 62:635–641, 1983

4. Massie MJ, Holland JC: Depression and the cancer patient. J Clin Psychiatry 51 (suppl):12–19, 1990

5. Watson M, Greer S, Rowden L, et al: Relationships between emotional control, adjustment to cancer and depression and anxiety in breast cancer patients. Psychol Med 21:51–57, 1991

6. Ron IG, Inbar MJ, Barak Y, et al: Organic delusional syndrome associated with tamoxifen treatment. Cancer 69:1415–1417, 1992

7. Jefferson JW: Tamoxifen-associated reduction in tricyclic antidepressant levels in blood (letter). J Clin Psychopharmacol 15:223–224, 1995

8. Spiegel D, Bloom JR, Kraemer HC, et al: Effect of psychosocial treatment on survival of patients with metastatic breast cancer. Lancet 2:888–891, 1989

APPENDIX:
SUPPORT GROUPS AND
ORGANIZATIONS

■ SUPPORT ORGANIZATIONS FOR INFERTILITY

RESOLVE, 1310 Broadway, Somerville, MA 02144-1731. Telephone, (617) 623-0744. National self-help organization for infertile couples. Sponsors support groups throughout the country to destigmatize the issue of infertility and enable couples to feel strengthened and less isolated. Telephone help line operates 9:00–12:00 A.M. and 1:00–4:00 P.M., Eastern Time, Mon. and Wed.–Fri.; 9:00–12:00 A.M. and 1:00–9:00 P.M., Eastern Time, Tues.; memberships available. Send SASE for further information.

■ SUPPORT ORGANIZATIONS FOR
POSTPARTUM DISORDERS

Postpartum Support International, 927 N. Kellogg Avenue, Santa Barbara, CA 93111. Telephone, (805) 967-7636. e-mail, 74442.3467@compuserve.com. An international network of individuals and organizations. Purpose is to increase awareness among public and professional communities about the emotional changes women often experience during pregnancy and after the birth of a baby.

■ CANCER SUPPORT GROUPS

Cancer Care, Inc., and the National Cancer Care Foundation, 1180 Avenue of the Americas, New York, NY 10036. Telephone, (212) 382-1955. Social service agency with specialized assistance for New York City residents and referrals to service agencies in areas outside or in New York.

Cancer Information Service. Telephone, 1-800-4-CANCER (422-6237). Telephone hotline for information on treatments and psychosocial resources.

CANCERVIVE, 6500 Wilshire Boulevard, Suite 500, Los Angeles, CA 90048. Telephone, (310) 203-9232. Group and individual counseling for women who are at least 6 months posttreatment. Newsletter publication.

National Alliance of Breast Cancer Organizations (NABCO), 9 East 37th Street, 10th Floor, New York, NY 10016. Telephone, (212) 719-0154. Fax, 212.719.0263. General information and referral resource. Quarterly newsletter publication.

The National Coalition for Cancer Survivorship, 1010 Wayne Avenue, Suite 500, Silver Spring, MD. Telephone, (301) 650-8868. National network of independent groups and individuals dedicated to providing support for cancer patients and their families.

Reach to Recovery. A program of the American Cancer Society. Telephone, 1-800-227-2345. Women who have had breast surgery (mastectomies with and without breast reconstruction or lumpectomies) visit and counsel women before and after their surgery.

We Can Weekend, Minneapolis, MN. Telephone, (612) 520-5211. Retreats for families dealing with cancer. Focus is on problems encountered by families affected by cancer. Designed for families with children and adolescents. Offered in many locations around the United States; the Minneapolis group will try to refer callers to a group in their area.

Y-ME National Association for Breast Cancer Information and Support, Inc., 18220 Harwood Avenue, Homewood, IL 60430. National toll-free telephone hotline, 1-800-221-2141, 9:00 A.M.–5:00 P.M. Central Time. 24-hour telephone, (312) 986-8228. Trained volunteers, most of them breast cancer survivors, provide information and support.

Index

Page numbers printed in **boldface** refer to tables or figures.